ORTHOPEDIC SECRETS

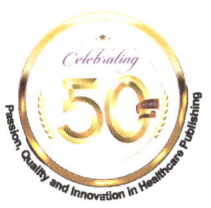

ORTHOPEDIC SECRETS

SECOND EDITION

Editor
DD Tanna MS (Ortho)
Mentor and Consulting Orthopedic Surgeon
Jaslok Hospital and Sir HN Reliance Hospital, Mumbai
Consulting Orthopedic Surgeon
Bhatia Hospital and Saifee Hospital, Mumbai
Ex-Professor
BYL Nair Hospital and TN Medical College
Mumbai University, Maharashtra, India

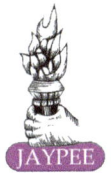

JAYPEE BROTHERS MEDICAL PUBLISHERS
The Health Sciences Publisher
New Delhi | London

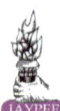

Jaypee Brothers Medical Publishers (P) Ltd.

Headquarters
Jaypee Brothers Medical Publishers (P) Ltd.
4838/24, Ansari Road, Daryaganj
New Delhi 110 002, India
Phone: +91-11-43574357
Fax: +91-11-43574314

Email: jaypee@jaypeebrothers.com

Overseas Office
JP Medical Ltd.
83, Victoria Street, London
SW1H 0HW (UK)
Phone: +44 20 3170 8910
Fax: +44 (0)20 3008 6180
E-mail: info@jpmedpub.com

Website: www.jaypeebrothers.com
Website: www.jaypeedigital.com

© 2020, Jaypee Brothers Medical Publishers

The views and opinions expressed in this book are solely those of the original contributor(s)/author(s) and do not necessarily represent those of editor(s) of the book.

All rights reserved. No part of this publication may be reproduced, stored or transmitted in any form or by any means, electronic, mechanical, photocopying, recording or otherwise, without the prior permission in writing of the publishers.

All brand names and product names used in this book are trade names, service marks, trademarks or registered trademarks of their respective owners. The publisher is not associated with any product or vendor mentioned in this book.

Medical knowledge and practice change constantly. This book is designed to provide accurate, authoritative information about the subject matter in question. However, readers are advised to check the most current information available on procedures included and check information from the manufacturer of each product to be administered, to verify the recommended dose, formula, method and duration of administration, adverse effects and contraindications. It is the responsibility of the practitioner to take all appropriate safety precautions. Neither the publisher nor the author(s)/editor(s) assume any liability for any injury and/or damage to persons or property arising from or related to use of material in this book.

This book is sold on the understanding that the publisher is not engaged in providing professional medical services. If such advice or services are required, the services of a competent medical professional should be sought.

Every effort has been made where necessary to contact holders of copyright to obtain permission to reproduce copyright material. If any have been inadvertently overlooked, the publisher will be pleased to make the necessary arrangements at the first opportunity. The **CD/DVD-ROM** (if any) provided in the sealed envelope with this book is complimentary and free of cost. **Not meant for sale**.

Inquiries for bulk sales may be solicited at: jaypee@jaypeebrothers.com

Orthopedic Secrets

First Edition: 2007

Second Edition: 2020

ISBN: 978-93-89188-448

Dedicated to

Trauma Society of India

Contributors

DD Tanna MS (Ortho)
Mentor and Consulting Orthopedic Surgeon
Jaslok Hospital and Sir HN Reliance Hospital, Mumbai
Consulting Orthopedic Surgeon
Bhatia Hospital and Saifee Hospital, Mumbai
Ex-Professor
BYL Nair Hospital and TN Medical College
Mumbai University, Maharashtra, India

RM Chandak MS (Ortho)
Director and Senior Consultant
Orthopedic Surgeon
Chandak Nursing Home
Nagpur, Maharashtra, India

Wasudeo Gadegone
MBBS MS (Gen Surg) MS (Ortho) MNAMS (Ortho) SICOT Fellow
Professor
Department of Orthopedics
Government Medical College
Chandrapur, Maharashtra, India

Preface to the Second Edition

Ward rounds were the ones which all my residents, including senior lecturers were apprehensive about. During those 4 hours of exhaustive, probing and hostile rounds, few weak hearted cried but never bunked. If they did, they knew, they would neither survive nor gain. During these rounds all of us got galvanized and read and thought about orthopedics and innovations. With our discussions, all of us got upgraded in orthopedics. This book is dedicated to all those who suffered those rounds with me and contributed to the growth of all of us. I am ever indebted to them, but definitely not sorry to have harass them...!!

This is a revised edition of the book *Orthopaedic Titbits*.

I am also thankful to all my fellows who have been patient during their time with me. They have also contributed profoundly in my thinking.

DD Tanna

Acknowledgments

I am thankful to my fellows Dr Sachin Yadav, Dr Chetan Satote and Dr Mohit Sharma to help me writing this 2nd edition. I also appreciate contributions from Dr RM Chandak, Nagpur; Dr Wasudeo Gadegone, Chandrapur, Maharashtra, Mumbai, Maharashtra, India.

I would like to thank Shri Jitendar P Vij (Group Chairman), Mr Ankit Vij (Managing Director), Ms Chetna Malhotra Vohra (Associate Director—Content Strategy) and M/s Nedup Denka Bhutia (Development Editor) of M/s Jaypee Brothers Medical Publishers (P) Ltd, New Delhi, India, for their untiring support during these two years.

Contents

1. **Day-to-day Problems** 1
   DD Tanna
   - Exercise Helps 1
   - Problem 1
   - Shoulder Mobilizing Exercises 3
   - Gait Correction 4
   - Seroma Collection 6
   - Procedure 7
   - Cerebrospinal Fluid Leak 8

2. **Bisphosphonate-induced Fractures** 9
   DD Tanna

3. **Out of Box Surgeries which has Worked in my Hands** 20
   DD Tanna

4. **Coccydynia** 33
   DD Tanna

5. **Comminuted Fracture** 41
   DD Tanna

6. **Distal Transverse Medial Malleolus Fracture** 52
   DD Tanna

7. **Head is Stronger than Machines (Investigations)** 58
   DD Tanna
   - Prolapsed Intervertebral Disc 58
   - Sternoclavicular Swelling 59
   - Synovial Herniation Pit of Femoral Neck 62
   - Acetabular Tuberculosis 67
   - Enchondroma of Femoral Head 69
   - Pain in Inguinal Area 73
   - Post-pregnancy Pain in Both Hips 79
   - Pain in Hip Unexplained 82
   - Infection after 15 years 82

8. Implant Removal 86
DD Tanna
- Austin Moore Removal 86
- Dynamic Hip Screw Removal 93
- Humerus Plate Removal 95
- Broken Nail Removal 96
- Broken Screw Removal 102

9. Interesting Cases 116
DD Tanna
- Case 1: Undisplaced Femur Neck Fracture 116
- Case 2: Conservative Treatment of
  Femur Neck Fracture 120
- Case 3: Waddling Gait 124
- Idiopathic Osteoporosis of Head of Femur 126
- Tip of Ulna Fracture 128

10. Intramedullary Fibula for Treatment of Nonunion Long Bones 136
DD Tanna
- Complications 162

11. Syndesmotic Injury and Ankle Fracture 168
DD Tanna

12. Posterior Malleolus 179
DD Tanna

13. Elbow Dislocation with Irreparable Fracture of Head of Radius 183
DD Tanna

14. Reamer/Irrigator/Aspirator (RIA) System: Use with induced Membrane to Fill-up Bone Defects 192
RM Chandak

15. J Nail Fixation for Surgical Neck Humerus Fractures in Elderly Osteoporotic Bones 202
RM Chandak
- Planning J nail Placement 206

- Case I 209
- Case II 210
- Case III 211

16. Screw Intramedullary Nail in Adult Forearm Fractures: New Concept 213
Wasudeo Gadegone
- The Design of the Screw Intramedullary Nail..............213
- Surgical Technique 214
- Pitfalls and Pearls 219

17. Humerus Nailing in Lateral Position 222
Wasudeo Gadegone
- Operative Technique 222
- Advantages of Lateral Position 228
- Pearls and Pitfalls 229

18. Screw Intramedullary Fixation of Displaced Clavicle Fractures.. 230
Wasudeo Gadegone
- Implant Design 230
- Step-by-step Description of Surgical Technique 231
- Advantages 234
- Pitfalls and Challenges 234

Index.. 237

Chapter 1

Day-to-day Problems

DD Tanna

EXERCISE HELPS

PROBLEM

Supination-pronation exercise is recommended for forearm and elbow fractures. Patient does not get in rhythm to do this, and moves wrist and fingers instead of the forearm.

Suggestion: By applying short wrist splint and semi-immobilizing the wrist, patient would be able to do supination and pronation exercises (Figs. 1.1A to D).

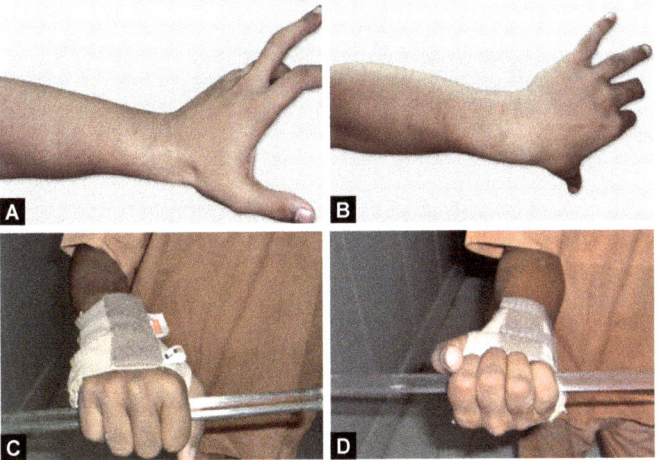

Figs. 1.1A to D: (A and B) Patient moves hand instead of moving of the forearm; (C and D) Proper supination and pronation exercise with short wrist splint.

When we ask patient to do ankle-mobilizing exercises after surgery, he tries to move only toe extensors and hence ankle is not exercised (Figs. 1.2A to C).

Suggestion: Strap the toes and he will do proper ankle exercises.

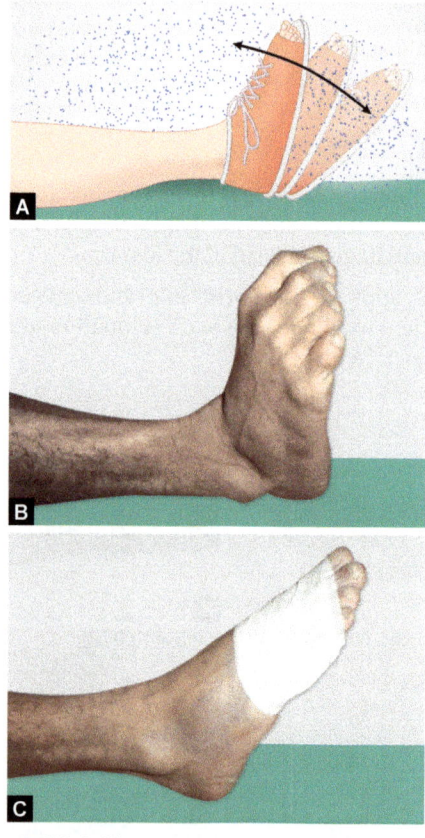

Figs. 1.2A to C: (A) Ankle exercises using shoe; (B) Trying to do ankle exercises but moving only toes; (C) By doing toe strapping.

SHOULDER MOBILIZING EXERCISES

Immobilize elbow with splint, so patient can do shoulder exercises better (Figs. 1.3A to C).

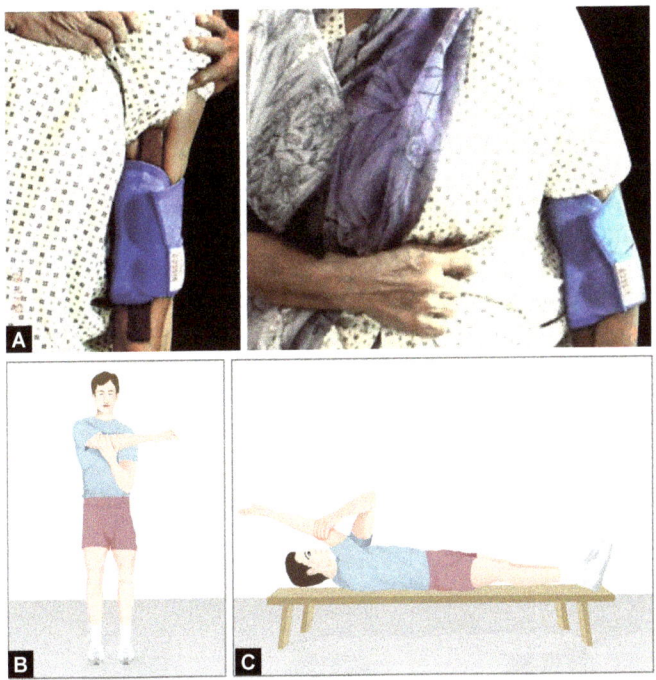

Figs. 1.3A to C: Shoulder exercises while immobilizing the elbow.

GAIT CORRECTION

After a long rehabilitation for injury or surgery of lower extremity, most of the patients walk with broad-based gait and find it difficult to correct this gait with conventional exercises. They can walk without pain. Fractures have already united and are pain free. They walk perfectly with stick on opposite side, but not on same side. They can walk without stick without pain but it is a hurried gait and broad base-like walking in a moving vehicle, in plane or on ship. This is typical of inability to walk perfectly due to loss of balancing.

When you ask him to stand on normal one leg stance, he can balance and stand straight. When he stands on affected one leg, he bends on opposite side to regain his balance but can stand without pain (Figs. 1.4A and B).

In this position if we give a stick to opposite hand, he can immediately stand straight without tilting on the opposite side (Fig. 1.4C). He should train himself when standing straight with stick in front of a mirror, and try to get balance and slowly reduce

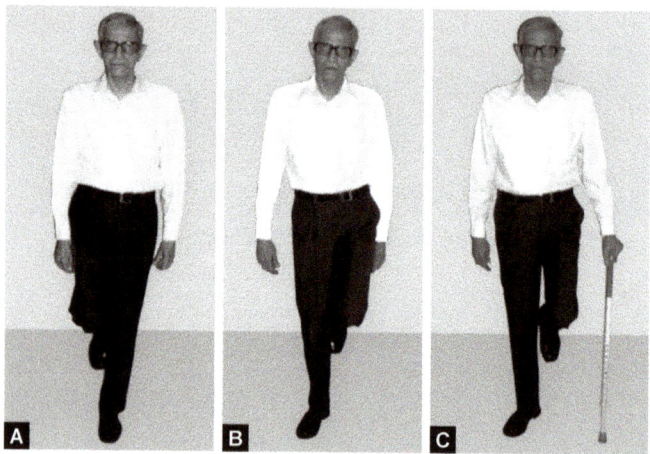

Figs. 1.4A to C: (A) Standing on normal leg; (B) Standing on the affected leg. Body turns on side to balance; (C) Body is straight if stick is on the opposite side.

the pressure on the stick, keeping the body straight, ultimately standing straight without stick.

Also, he should be trained to walk in a straight line and should walk on one tile on the floor, with equal steps, without steps going on the other tile, avoiding unequal hurried steps.

This will allow him to relearn the balance and he will be able to walk straight. This has been very well written by George Perkins in his book of reminisces many years back.

Suggestion: Do pay attention toward gait training of the patient after long convalescence (Figs. 1.5A to E).

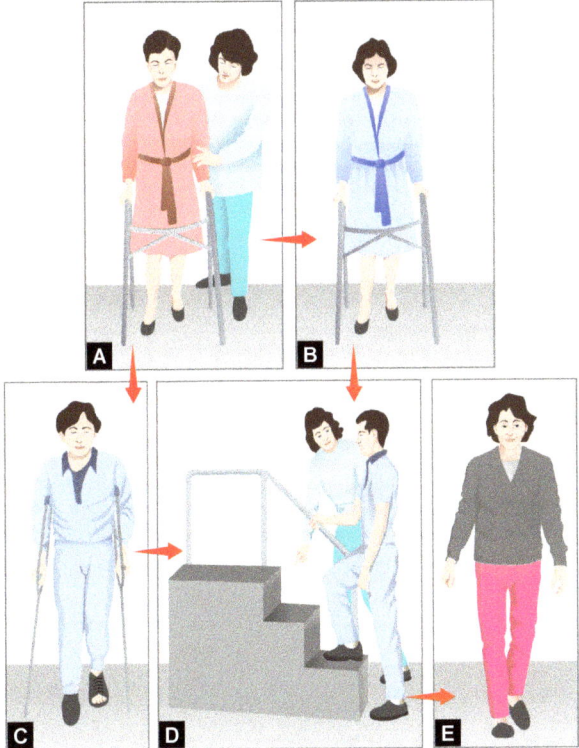

Figs. 1.5A to E: Gait training.

SEROMA COLLECTION

Blunt injury with hematoma formation in soft tissue (Fig. 1.6) results in serum exudates after 1 week, and is difficult to treat. After aspiration, it fills up again and this is due to dead space remaining in the area after aspiration, which refills in short time.

Suggestion: I suggest to put vacuum drainage and allow the cavity to collapse for 3/4 days. Enough adhesions form between the layers of the seroma cavity, and dead space will be obliterated, avoiding seroma formation again.

My suggestion is, put the tube in before aspiration so that placing of the tube is perfect when fluid is inside. It may end up in an empty cavity if introduced after seroma is evacuated and then tried to introduce in collapsed space.

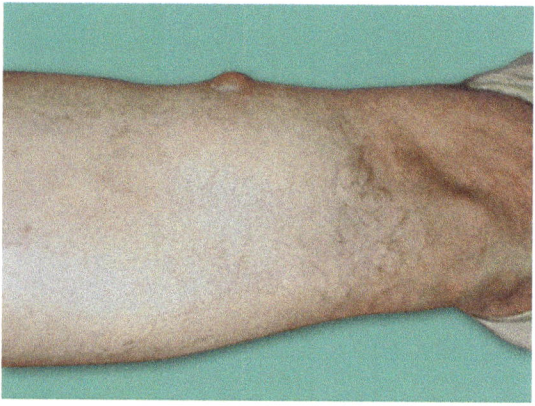

Fig. 1.6: Hematoma after blunt injury, 10 days old with a small blister on the hematoma.

PROCEDURE (FIGS. 1.7A TO D)

On palpation, dependent part is localized and a triple trocar (used for external fixation) is pierced into the swelling. Do not drain the serum after confirming the correct cavity. Now remove trocar and keep outer hollow tube and confirm the patency. Introduce an 8 mm drainage tube in this sleeve and connect it to the vacuum bottle with negative suction after removing the hollow outer tube. Keep this negative suction bottle tied up on patient's extremity for 3 days and allow him to walk about.

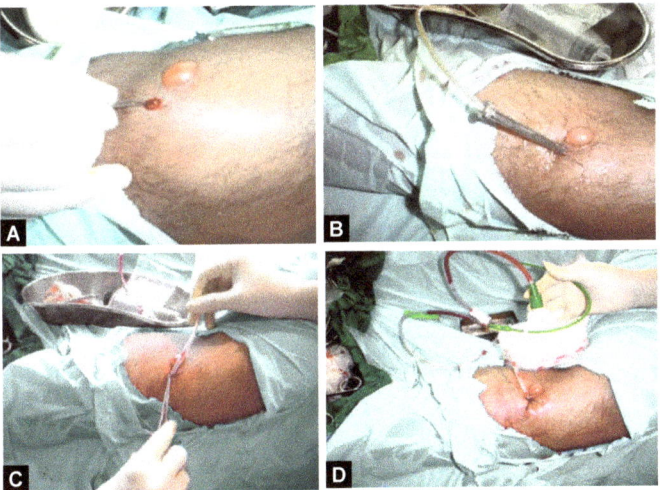

Figs. 1.7A to D: Suction drainage of seroma cavity.

CEREBROSPINAL FLUID LEAK

Cerebrospinal fluid (CSF) leaks, after major missed dural tears or unsuccessful repairs, can be treated by "Proximal CSF diversion" by passing an intradural catheter at a level higher than the dural tear level. Pass lumbar puncture needle and on confirmation of CSF, pass a catheter used for epidural, through this needle and then remove the needle, confirm CSF flow, and attach it to a sterile dependent (not negative suction) drain bottle. In 3/4 days, dural tear would have healed as CSF is now bypassed proximally leaving the leak area to dry and to close. Catheter can then be pulled out. Supportive treatment of head low position, plenty of fluids, and tablet acetazolamide (Diamox) and complete bed rest, for whatever it is worth, are given.

Bisphosphonate-induced Fractures

Chapter 2

DD Tanna

According to the American Society for Bone and Mineral Research (ASBMR), bisphosphonate-induced fractures are atypical femoral fractures after prolonged use of bisphosphonate. This can be seen anywhere between the subtrochanteric to supracondylar femur level. A bilateral involvement is very commonly seen. Patient does not give history of any trauma. Theoretically, bisphosphonates suppress bone turnover and thus might be associated with accumulated microdamage in bone. The fracture is either transverse or short oblique in configuration and start off as incomplete fracture involving the lateral cortex (Fig. 2.1). In contrast to this, the insufficiency fractures are located over the medial femoral cortex.

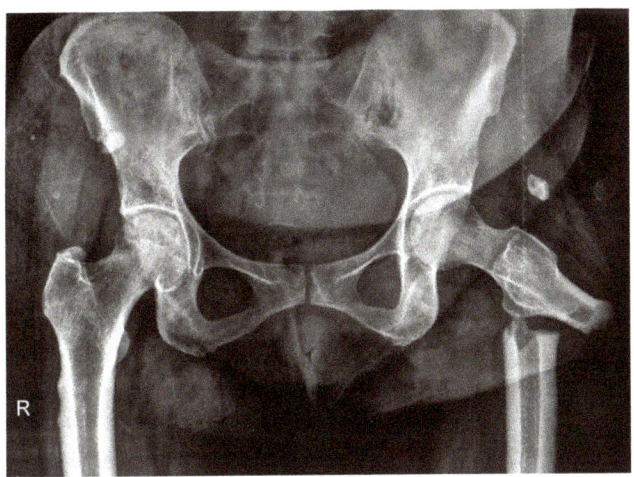

Fig. 2.1: Transverse fracture seen at subtrochanteric level (left side). Observe the lateral cortex thickening (right side).

Patient having history of prolonged bisphosphonate intake presents with complaints of pain and discomfort over proximal thigh. Here again remember, *X-ray of both hips and upper two-thirds thigh is essential.* In the earlier stages, they appear only as cortical thickening over lateral aspect of the proximal femur (Figs. 2.2A and B). This cortical thickening (one of the minor radiographic features) is believed to result from an impaired ability of bone to remodel because of prolonged bisphosphonate use, leading to an accumulation of microdamage and compromised bone strength. If not appreciated on the X-ray, a high index of suspicion should still be maintained. Magnetic resonance imaging (MRI) or positron emission tomography–computed tomography (PET-CT) scan comes to the rescue for diagnosis in these situations (Figs. 2.3A and B). MRI and bone scanning have greater sensitivity than radiography for an incipient stress fracture diagnosis. When the fracture is in the incipient, impending stage, and has not yet developed, PET-CT is the most sensitive test to diagnose it

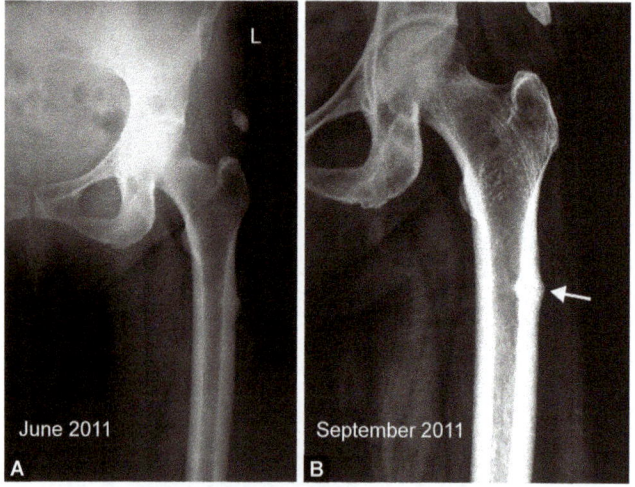

Figs. 2.2A and B: Fracture begins as lateral cortex thickening. A 60-year-old on osteofos administration for 6 years.

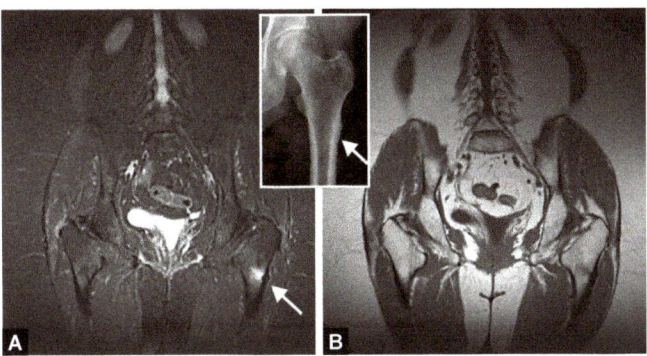

Figs. 2.3A and B: Incipient stage fracture picked up on MRI.

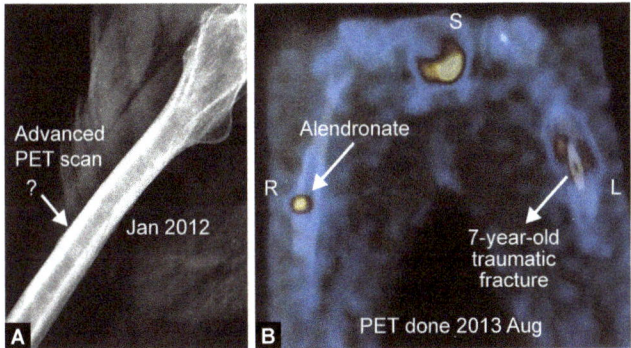

Figs. 2.4A and B: PET-CT diagnoses this fracture even when the MRI is negative.

(Figs. 2.4A and B). If a fracture is detected at this stage and treated early, all future nonunions can be avoided. These fractures are not so cruel if diagnosed early. If treated at the incipient stage, a simple interlock nailing in intact femur is all that is needed (Figs. 2.5A and B).

These fractures are notorious for delayed union and nonunion if not treated properly. Bone biopsies in these patients showed evidence of severely suppressed bone turnover and

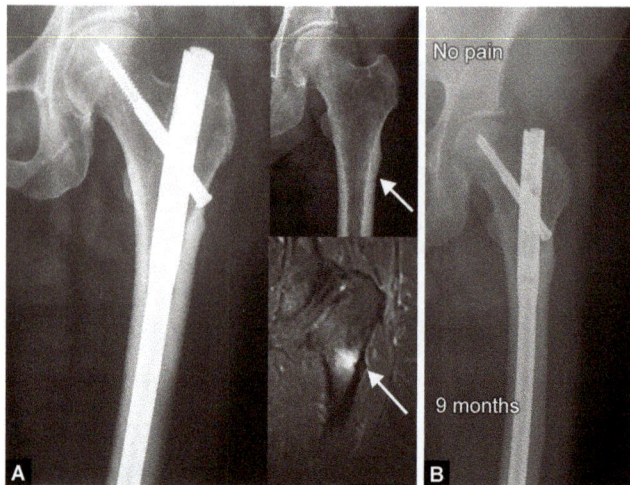

Figs. 2.5A and B: Fracture heals well if nailed in the early stages.

fracture healing that was delayed or absent. Hence they should be nailed and not plated as far as possible (Figs. 2.6 and 2.7). Injection teriparatide and local ultrasound therapy should be started from Day 1 to enhance chances of healing. In management of nonunion, nails are augmented with plating to achieve rigid fixation. Whether auto bone graft is useful in this particular case is questionable, because the auto graft is itself bisphosphonate affected. Hence, I prefer to use bone morphogenetic protein (BMP), if at all the need arises.

So the take-home messages here are:
- Incipient fractures should be diagnosed early with MRI or PET-CT scan to avoid its progression to complete fracture and its complications of delayed union or nonunion.
- A patient with history of bisphosphonate intake for long-term and pain in upper end femur should always be investigated.
- Intramedullary implant is always preferred, as these fracture take long time to heal.

Chapter 2: Bisphosphonate-induced Fractures

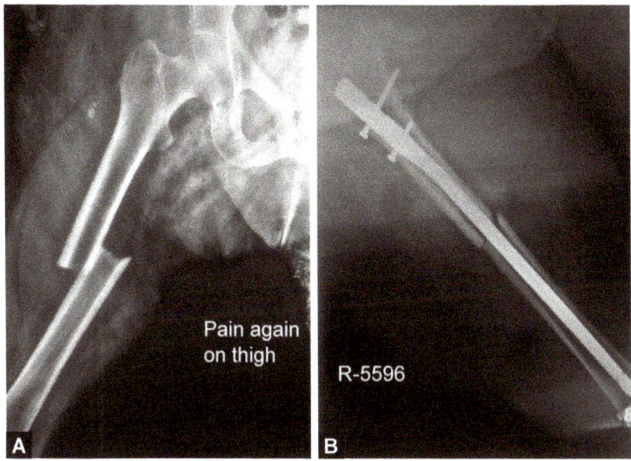

Figs. 2.6A and B: Interlock nailing is preferred rather than plating for these fractures.

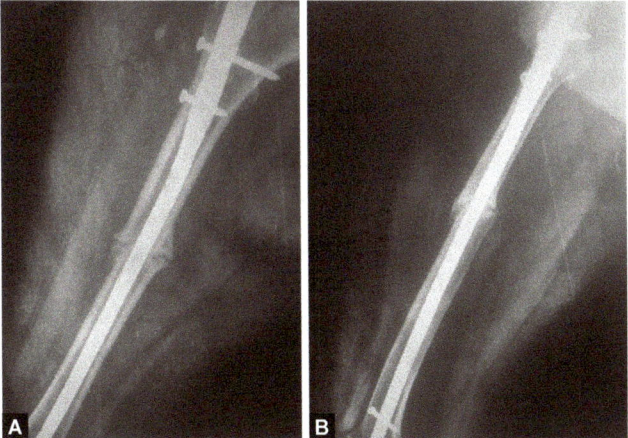

Figs. 2.7A and B: Healing fractures.

- In view of the high frequency of bilateral involvement, imaging of the contralateral femoral shaft with X-rays, MRI, or an isotope bone scan should be performed. MRI and bone scanning have greater sensitivity than radiography for an incipient stress fracture.

So now the question posed is—with all these complications and risks, is it worthwhile to give bisphosphonates to patients? According to the ASBMR taskforce, these fractures are seen in 2 cases per 1 lakh patients on 2 years of use and 78 cases per 1 lakh on 7 years of use. Recommendation is to give for 3–5 years and then give a drug holiday to the patient.

I would like to mention a difficult case related to alendronate therapy I came across.

An 85-year-old Indian woman was presented with swelling and tenderness around left proximal femur after trivial trauma during walking at her home. She was not able to bear weight on left lower limb. On enquiry, she was on alendronate therapy for past 6 years. She did not give any specific history of any prodromal thigh pain. She had been operated for bilateral total knee replacement in the past which was fine on examination. There were no bruises around the thigh, no neurovascular deficit, and pulses were strong. On X-ray, there was a simple two part low subtrochanteric transverse fracture (Figs. 2.8A and B).

All her blood tests were normal. The patient was subjected to below knee traction. After her medical fitness, she was taken up for surgery on 4th day of fracture and intramedullary nailing was planned for her. Increased medial cortex density on X-ray was missed, as shown in Figures 2.8A and B, before surgery. After spinal anesthesia, 4 cm incision was made proximal to greater trochanter in line with shaft. The greater trochanter was located with guidewire and entry was made through the tip of trochanter under fluoroscopic guidance. Proximal reamer was used to open the canal. But we were unable to proceed the guidewire distally as shown in Figure 2.9. We tried repeatedly with awl to make the proximal entry large and then tried to insert the guidewire. Because of our repeated attempts

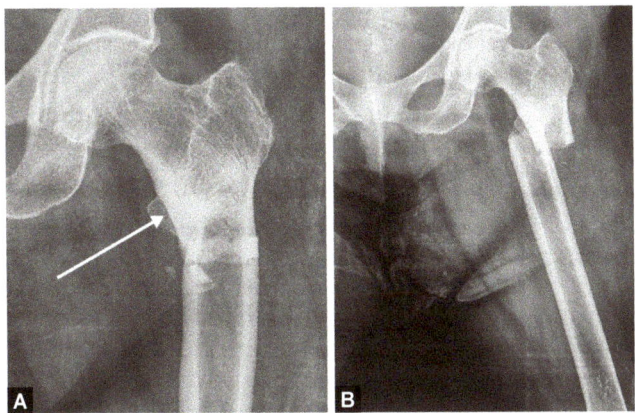

Figs. 2.8A and B: X-ray showing transverse fracture of subtrochanteric area. There is medial cortical thickening (arrow).

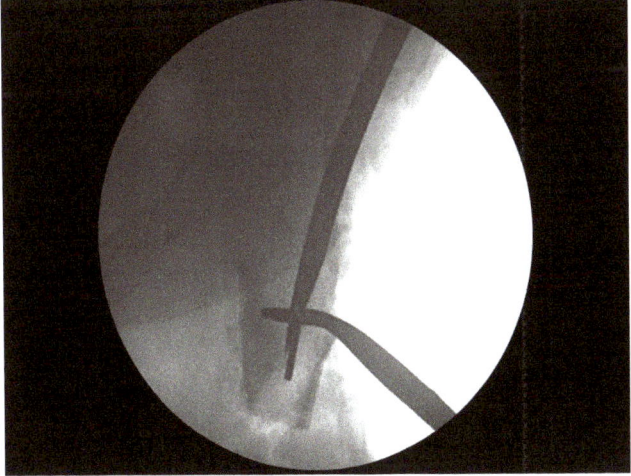

Fig. 2.9: C-arm image showing obliteration of canal and inability to pass guidewire into distal part of fracture.

and osteoporosis, there could have been some unnoticed undisplaced cracks which occurred on anterior, posterior, and lateral walls of proximal femur. Then the decision to explore the fracture site was taken. Obliteration of proximal canal by dense sclerotic bone was observed. The medullary canal was recreated with small drills with utmost care until reamers can be passed from the fracture end proximally as shown in Figures 2.10A and B. The consistency of obliteration was even harder or equal to cortical bone. Then while inserting the long A2FN Nail, we encountered the split in posterior and lateral walls of proximal segment as shown in Figure 2.11.

Then we did the encirclage wiring to hold the fragments and once the fragments were in place, we inserted the guidewire into the neck and then the lag screw was inserted as shown in Figures 2.12A and B. After insertion of lag screw, one more encirclage wiring was done to give extra hold. Allo bone grafting was done after distal locking. Final C-arm pictures were satisfactory as shown in Figures 2.13A and B. Immediate postoperative and 3 month follow-up X-rays are shown in Figures 2.14A and B.

There are several cases reported of alendronate fractures but there is only a single case report on canal obliteration due to prolonged alendronate therapy and subsequent difficulty

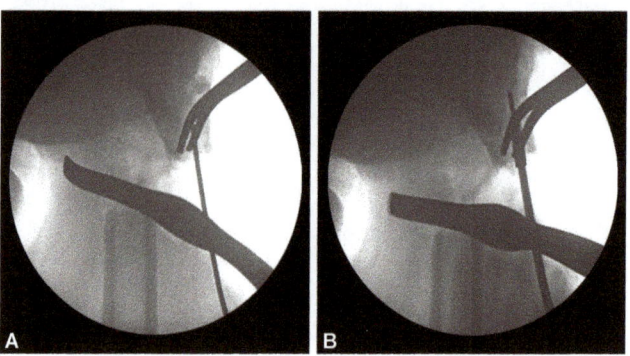

Figs. 2.10A and B: Opening of blocked medullary canal from fracture end with drill bits and reamer.

Chapter 2: Bisphosphonate-induced Fractures 17

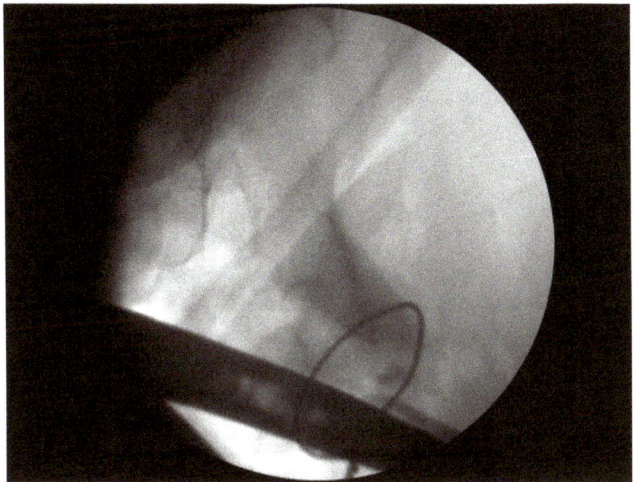

Fig. 2.11: Lateral view showing fractured posterior wall which is held together by encirclage wiring.

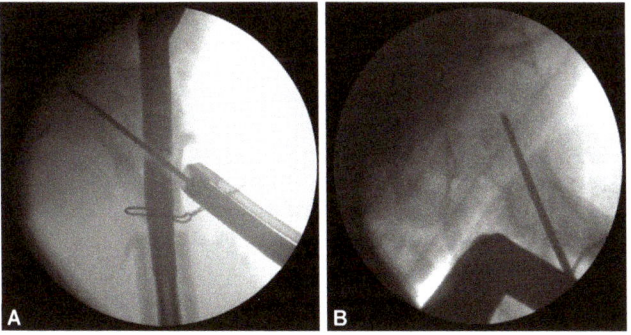

Figs. 2.12A and B: X-ray anteroposterior and lateral views showing guidewire insertion in neck.

in nailing or iatrogenic fracture. Femoral canal obliteration secondary to prolonged alendronate use, a case report by Chin Tat Lim et al. from National University Hospital, Singapore.

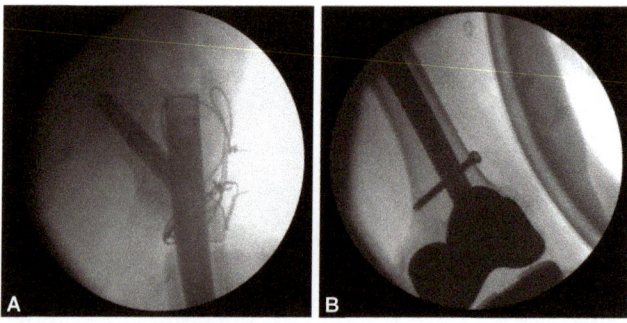

Figs. 2.13A and B: Final C-arm images—anteroposterior view.

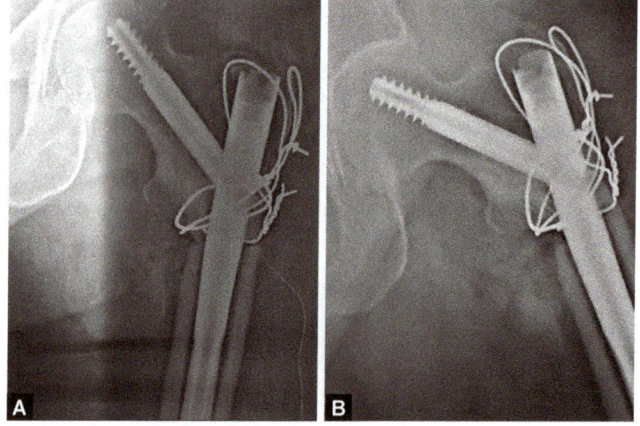

Figs. 2.14A and B: (A) Day 1 postoperative X-ray anteroposterior view; (B) Three months follow-up X-ray.

In our patient due to the prolonged alendronate therapy, there was inhibition of bone remodelling which resulted in dense sclerotic cortical bone which obliterated medullary canal. We missed it preoperatively and after repeated unsuccessful attempts to put guidewire, we realized about the obliterated medullary canal. Then the medullary canal was approached from the fracture end and canal was recreated with small drill bits and then reamers. Due to the associated osteoporosis, while inserting final nail, we encountered fracture of posterior and lateral proximal femur walls which was treated with encircle wiring and bone grafting.

SUGGESTED READING

1. Lim CT, Setiobudi T, Das De S. Femoral canal obliteration secondary to prolonged alendronate use: a case report. J Orthop Surg (Hong Kong). 2012;20(1):115-7.

Out of Box Surgeries which has Worked in my Hands

Chapter 3

DD Tanna

These are few surgeries and steps which are probably not evidence based. I have done, and succeeded in my hands, which I am presenting here.

- *Nailing with interfragmentary screws:*

  I will quote a few examples to get this through.

  A 72-year-old male with long oblique fracture of upper third shaft of humerus is presented (Figs. 3.1A to C). Fracture is reduced by anterior lateral approach, opening the fracture ends. The fracture is accurately reduced, held with large bone holding clamps. Entry portal is made in the head for standard

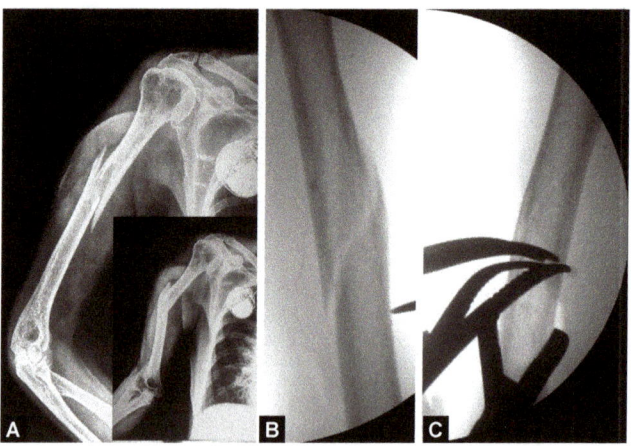

Figs. 3.1A to C: Long oblique proximal humerus fracture, open reduction, and held by bone holding clamps.

humerus interlocking nail. After reaming to adequate size and depth, nail is introduced and proximally locking screws are inserted. Then interfragmentary screws (2.5 mm) are drilled perpendicular to the fracture bypassing the nail. Screws of appropriate size are inserted. Usually requires minimum two screws for adequate compression (Figs. 3.2 to 3.6).

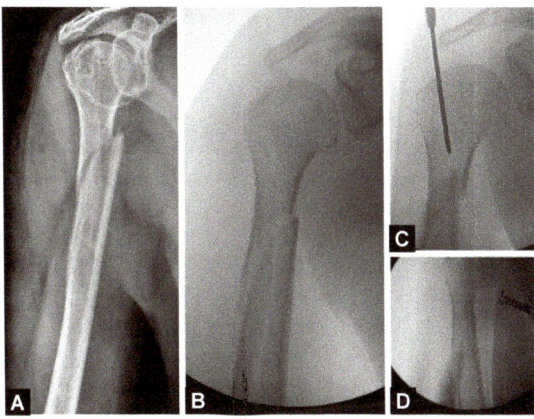

Figs. 3.2A to D: Initial closed reduction C-arm images.

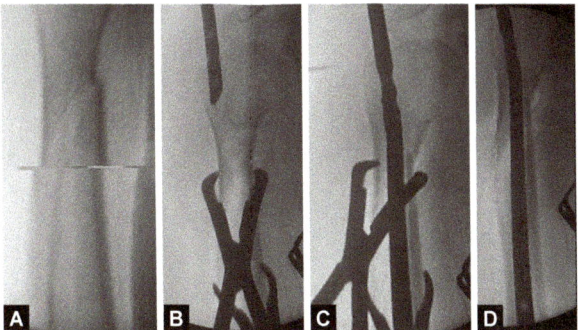

Figs. 3.3A to D: Fracture is reduced first, and held with clamps, before passing the nail.

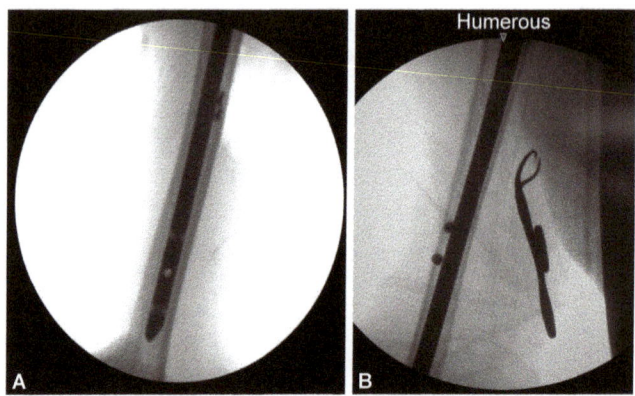

Figs. 3.4A and B: Interlock nailing done, interfragmentary screw put at the fracture site bypassing the nail.

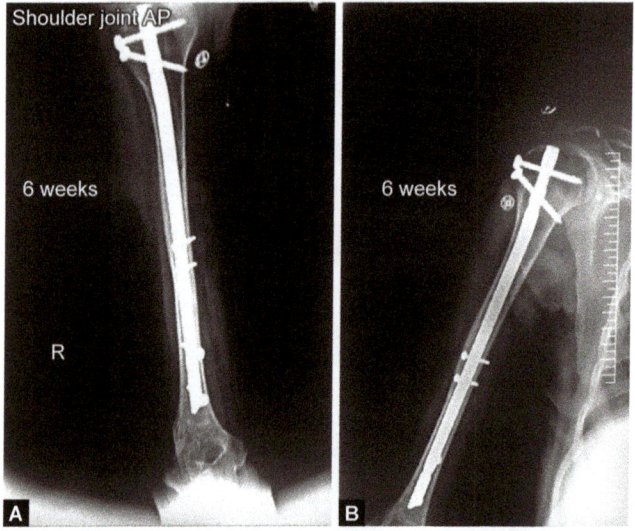

Figs. 3.5A and B: Six weeks follow-up X-rays show near complete union.

Chapter 3: Out of Box Surgeries which has Worked in my Hands 23

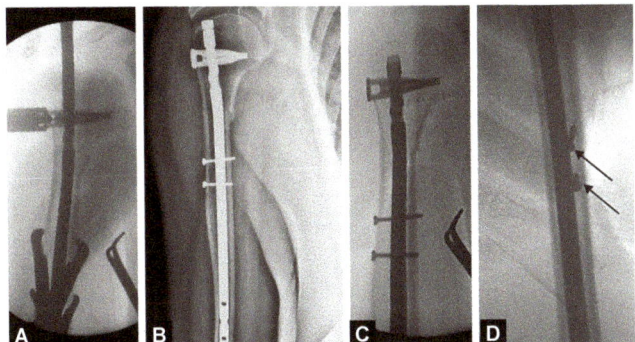

Figs. 3.6A to D: Similar 2nd case is presented.

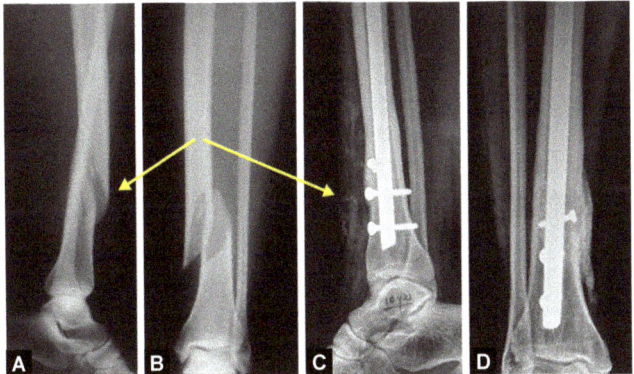

Figs. 3.7A to D: Open reduction, interlock nailing and interfragmentary screws at fracture site.

Similar technique can be used for open reduction, nailing, and interfragmentary screw fixation in long oblique kind of shaft fracture of long bones like femur, tibia as depicted in the images below (Figs. 3.7 to 3.11).

24 | Orthopedic Secrets

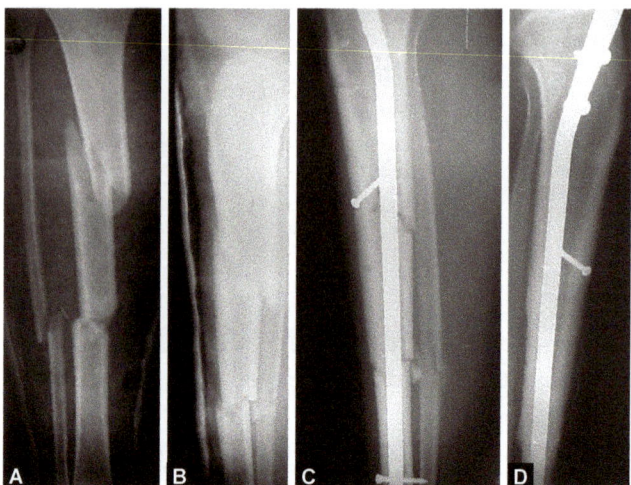

Figs. 3.8A to D: Similar thing is done for segmental fracture tibia. Fracture is reduced, held with clamps, and nailed, before lag screw is put.

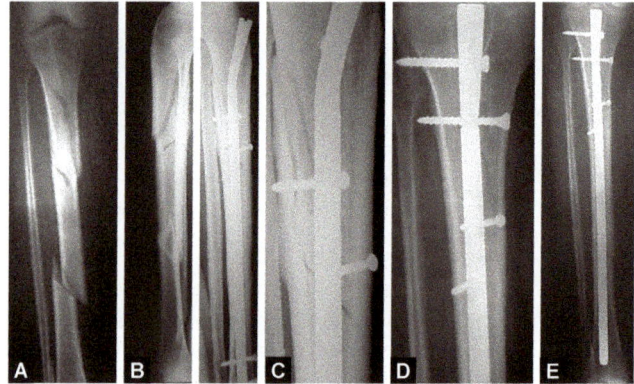

Figs. 3.9A to E: Lag screw of upper fragment to get anatomical position.

Chapter 3: Out of Box Surgeries which has Worked in my Hands

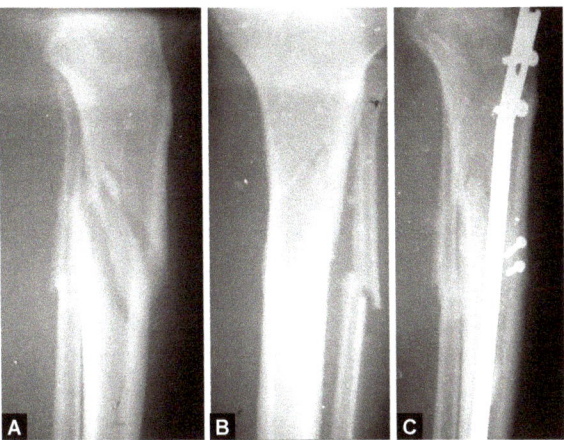

Figs. 3.10A to C: Interfragmentary screw and nail in long oblique fracture.

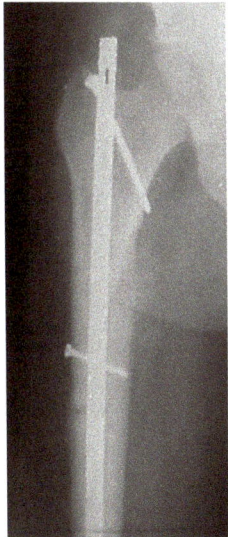

Fig. 3.11: Fracture shaft femur treated with interlocking nail. The butterfly fragment is reduced and fixed with interfragmentary screw.

- While doing uncemented hemiarthroplasty for treatment of comminuted intertrochanteric fracture or even for nonunion intertrochanteric (IT) fracture, we encountered a wide metaphyseal area. Most of the uncemented prosthesis designs do not give adequate stability in this metaphyseal region. I used two methods to compensate here.
  1. The femur neck is osteotomized out of the head extracted and can be used as a corticocancellous graft between the prosthesis and the metaphyseal cortex (Figs. 3.12 to 3.14).
  2. The second method I adopt is using cement to augment and broaden the part of the prosthesis which will sit in the metaphyseal region (Fig. 3.15). Both these methods give additional rotational stability to the prosthesis.
     - Of late, I have been, fixing, anatomically reduced, avulsed lesser trochanter, with cerclage wires. This gives, the shape of the neck similar, to transcervical fracture. This makes it easy to find version during replacement of the IT fracture as in Figures 3.14C and D. I also add hook plate, to control, greater trochanter (GT), healing

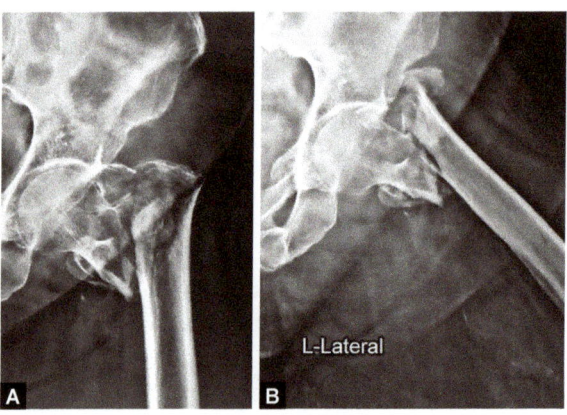

Figs. 3.12A and B: Highly comminuted intertrochanteric fracture, suitable for a hemiarthroplasty rather than fixation.

Chapter 3: Out of Box Surgeries which has Worked in my Hands

with the bone. Nonunion of the avulsed GT is a known complication of replacement in trochanteric fracture replacement.

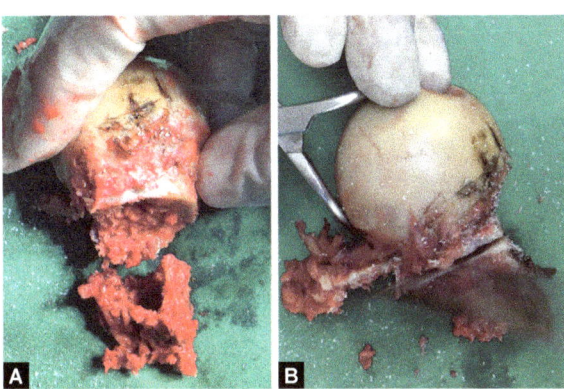

Figs. 3.13A and B: Femur neck osteotomized from the neck extracted while doing the hemiarthroplasty.

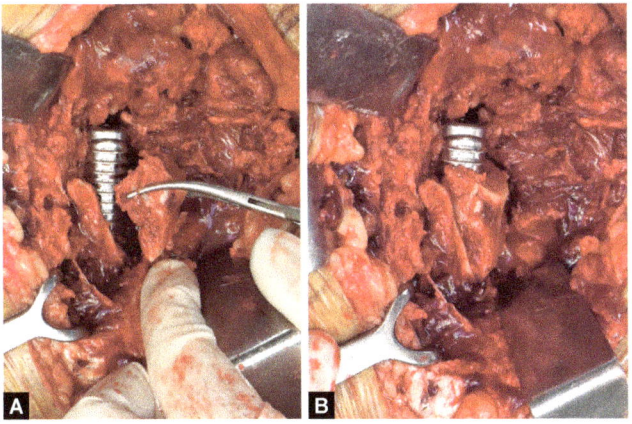

Figs. 3.14A to B

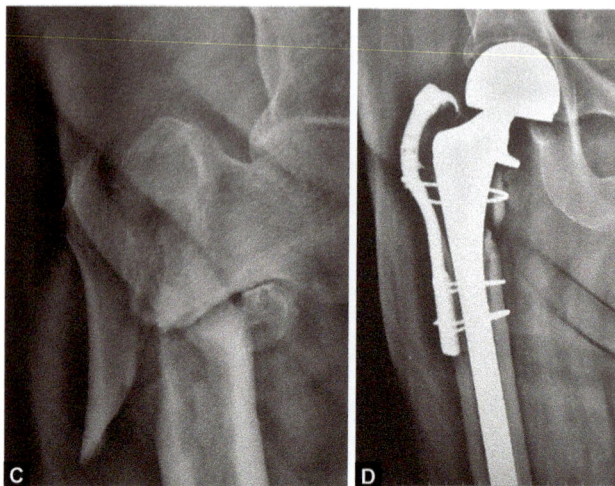

Figs. 3.14C to D

Figs. 3.14A to D: Osteotomized neck is used as a corticocancellous graft in the metaphyseal region for rotational stability.

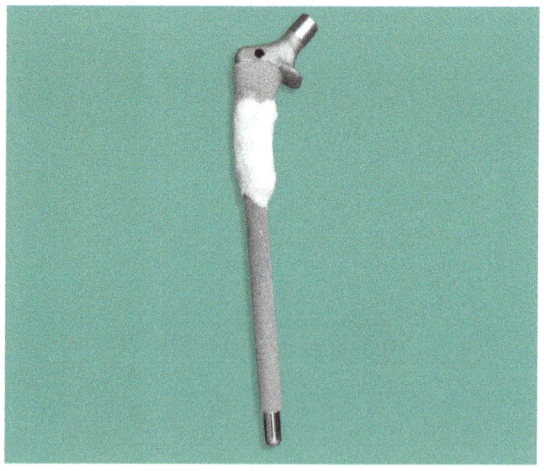

Fig. 3.15: Cement used to augment the metaphyseal area of the prosthesis.

- In supracondylar femur fracture requiring double plating or in periprosthetic fractures of distal femur, there is no consensus on the implant to be used on the medial femoral condyle. The implant I found most suitable and fits very well is the standard PHILOS plate used in the proximal humerus fracture fixation. It gives option for multiple locking screws in the femoral condyle with good stability (Figs. 3.16 to 3.18).
- While treating nonunion of fractures where we want to fix the fracture with a nail and a plate, it becomes very difficult to fix the plate due to the nail inside the medullary cavity. Bicortical screws are desired for stability but difficult, to execute. Unicortical locking screws can be used but they are not very reliable for adequate stability. The method I follow is to use a 3.5 mm screw with washer in a 4.5 mm hole. The 2.5 mm drill is used to make the hole obliquely anterior or

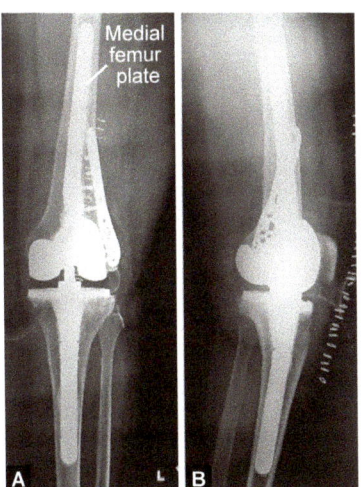

Figs. 3.16A and B: Fixing accidental supracondylar femur fracture while doing total knee replacement (TKR) or supracondylar fracture requiring double plating, PHILOS plate is good implant for medial plating.

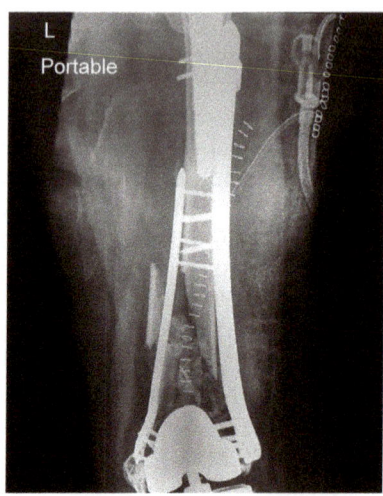

Fig. 3.17: Proximal humerus locking plate fits well on medial femur condyl.

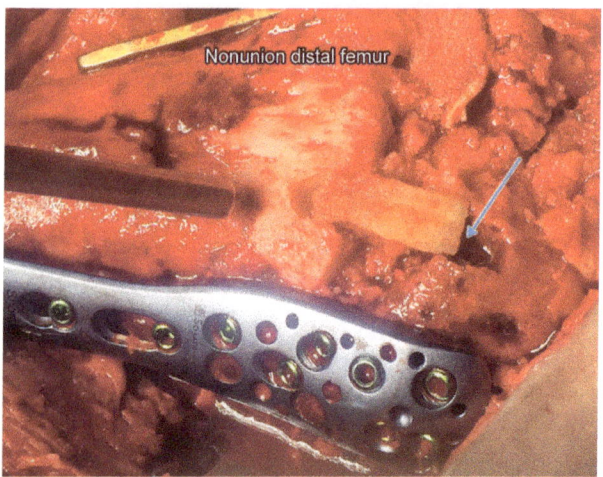

Figs. 3.18: Nonunion distal femur, proximal humerus PHILOS plate on medial side, fits well.

posterior to the nail. Once the 3.5 mm bicortical purchase is achieved, it gives a nice stable hold and the required rigidity for nonunion fracture healing (Figs. 3.19 and 3.20).

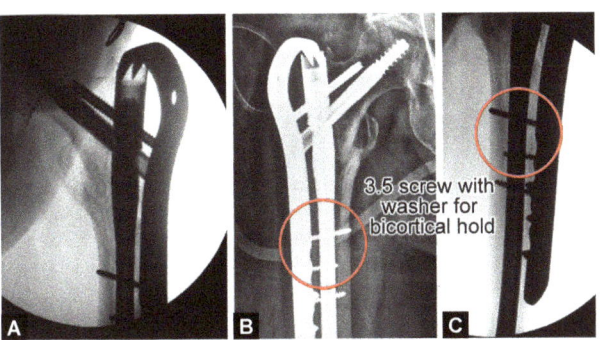

Fig. 3.19A to C: (A) Nonunion intertrochanteric fracture treated with proximal femur hook plate; (B and C) 3.5 mm cortical screw with washer used to get bicortical purchase bypassing the intramedullary nail.

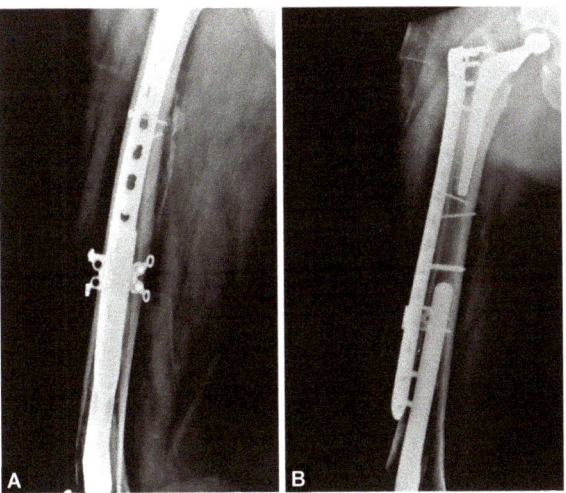

Figs. 3.20A and B: Such Saddle plate with extension, to put screws on the side of the nail is also available.

- While doing replacement for IT fracture, wiring of trochanter often fails and trochanter does not unite and retracts out. I use hook plate to fix comminuted trochanter, which maintains trochanter in position (Figs. 3.21 and 3.22).

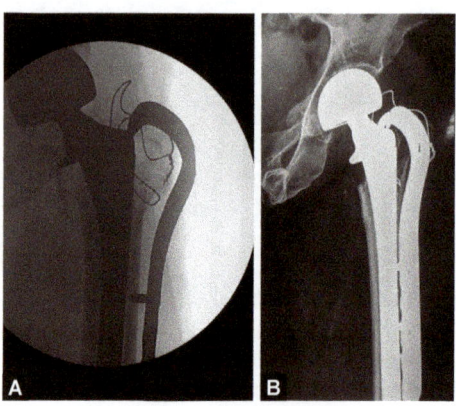

Figs. 3.21A and B: Hook plate used to fix greater trochanter.

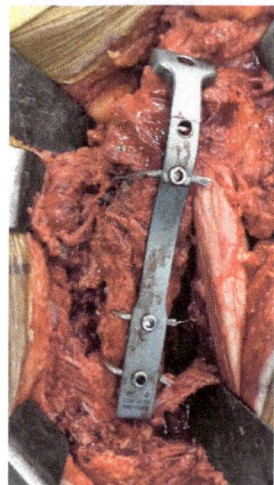

Fig. 3.22: Intraoperative photograph of the hook plate.

Chapter 4

Coccydynia

DD Tanna

Pain in coccyx is very troublesome at times. Soft cushion is the only possible treatment advised, which partially works. Fortunately most often pain in coccyx subsides over a due course of time and needs no further treatment. It is seen more often after delivery and after a fall on stairs and landing on buttocks (Figs. 4.1A and B). One must be careful in diagnosis, as it is presented often as a disguised pilonidal sinus.

- Most of the coccydynia subside with time, all they need is a soft cushion for sitting (Fig. 4.2). They get more pain on leaning backward (Figs. 4.3A to C). There is hypothesis that in flexion, there is abnormal dural tension, which is relieved on extension, probably the reason why transrectal manipulation works (Fig. 4.4). Pain on sitting on hard surface, no pain on standing or sleeping. Local steroid is not

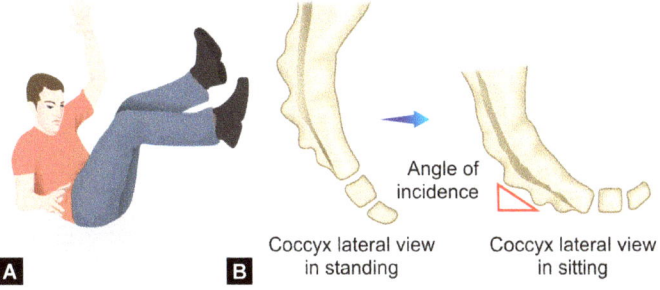

Figs. 4.1A and B: (A) Fall on buttocks gives fracture of coccyx; (B) Angulation of coccyx.

34 *Orthopedic Secrets*

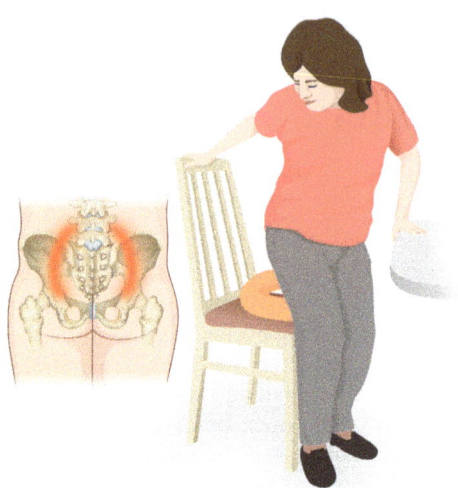

Fig. 4.2: Use soft cushion while sitting.

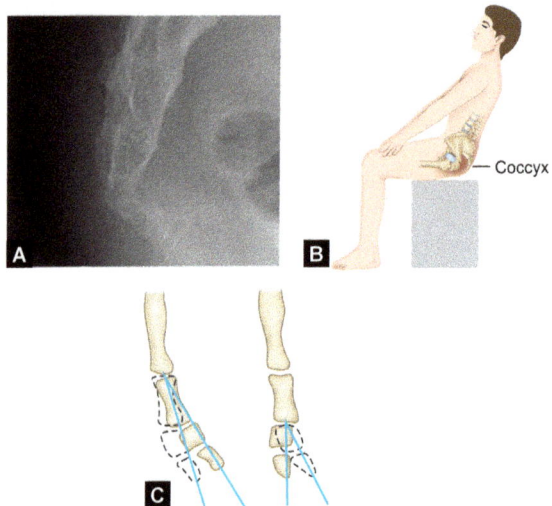

Figs. 4.3A to C: (A) Injury of coccyx; (B) More pain on leaning backward; (C) Movements of coccyx on leaning give pain.

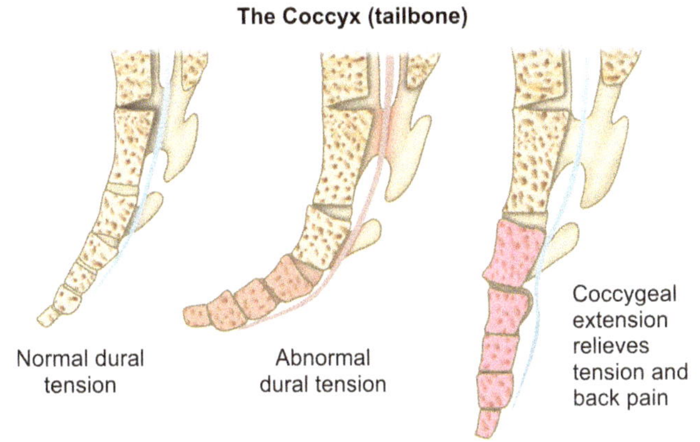

The Coccyx (tailbone)

| Normal dural tension | Abnormal dural tension | Coccygeal extension relieves tension and back pain |

Fig. 4.4: Abnormal dural tension on flexion of coccyx. Probably the reason why transrectal manipulation works.

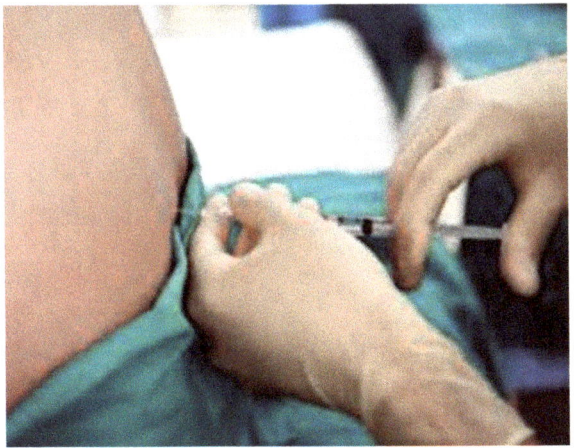

Fig. 4.5: Some people claim, local injection gives relief, I feel chances of infection are higher in this area, I never do it.

helpful and may give local infection; I never do it (Fig. 4.5). Recalcitrant cases do need excision of coccyx. Before going for surgery, wait for a year, for pain to settle down. Most will

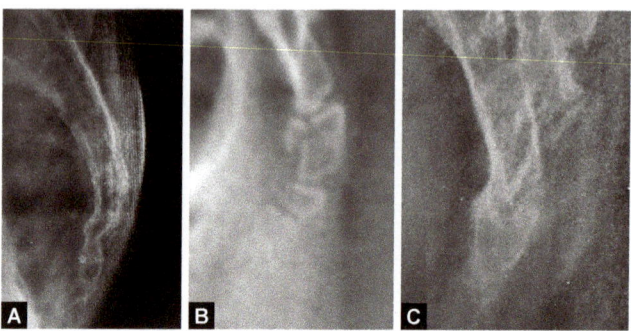

Figs. 4.6A to C: Most will settle down in about 1 year time.

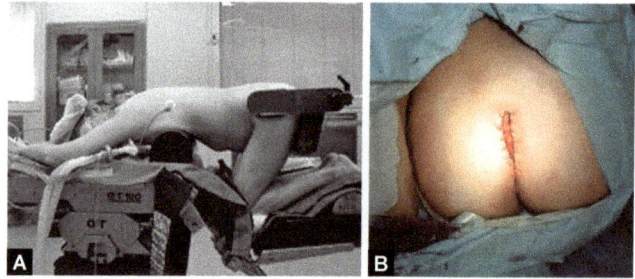

Figs. 4.7A and B: Knee chest position—two views.

be ok in 1 year (Figs. 4.6A to C). If still uncomfortable, excision of coccyx is a possible way forward. Surgery of excision of coccyx is done in knee-chest position (Figs. 4.7A and B). Adrenaline injection is used to improve vision. Remain on bone in center before injection, do not stray on side of bone. Cut the skin and go up to bone, remaining all along on the bone. Remove periosteum and feel the bone. One can see

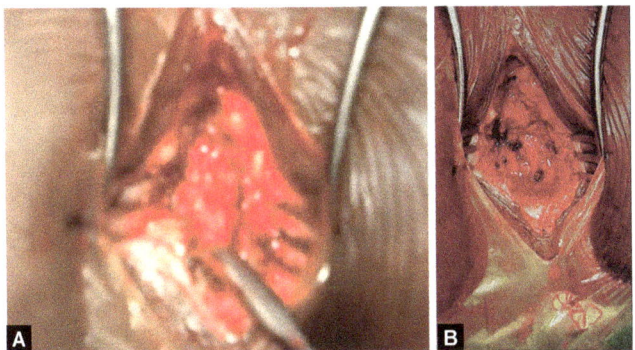

Figs. 4.8A and B: After exposure, movements of the loose piece of coccyx can be felt.

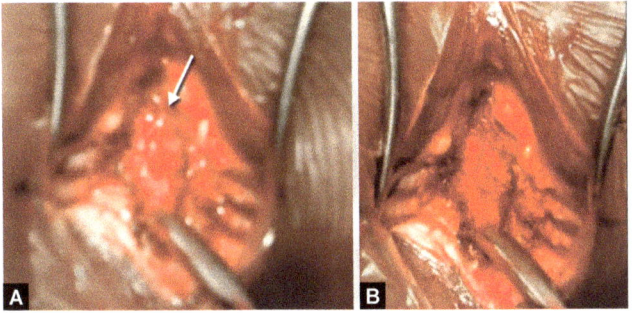

Figs. 4.9A and B: Movements at pseudo-joint, enter from this space (arrow).

the area of movements between two pieces of coccyx (Figs. 4.8A and B). Enter this area from the proximal side, hold the coccyx with towel, clip, and create a space between bone and soft tissue, anterior to the coccyx bone, hugging the bone all the time to avoid injury to rectum (Figs. 4.9 to 4.13).

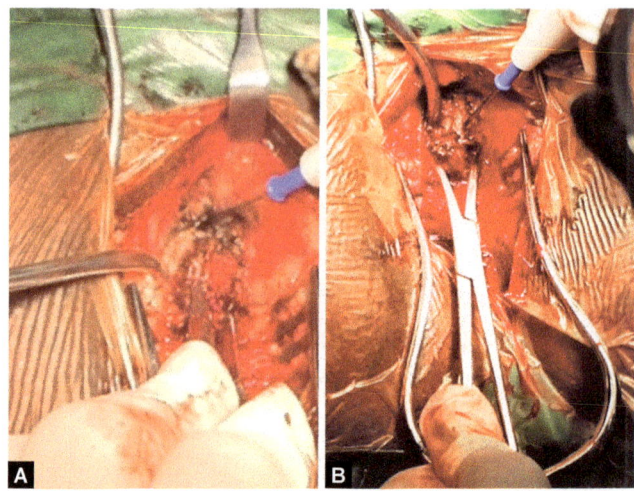

Figs. 4.10A and B: Hold with towel clip and clear this piece all around, hugging the bone to avoid injury to rectum.

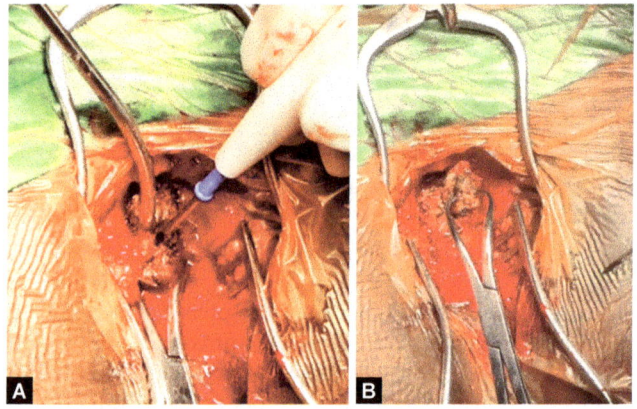

Figs. 4.11A and B: Dissection around bone. Excised coccyx in towel clip.

Chapter 4: Coccydynia

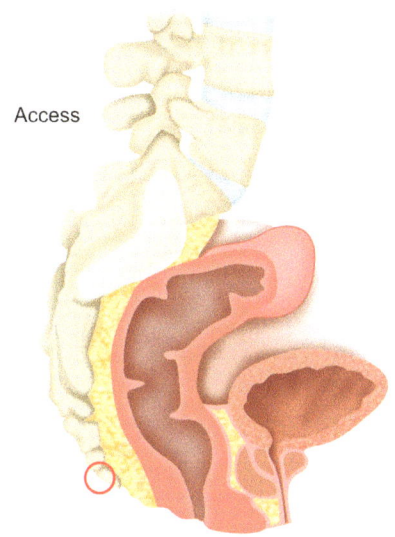

Fig. 4.12: Rectum is nearby.

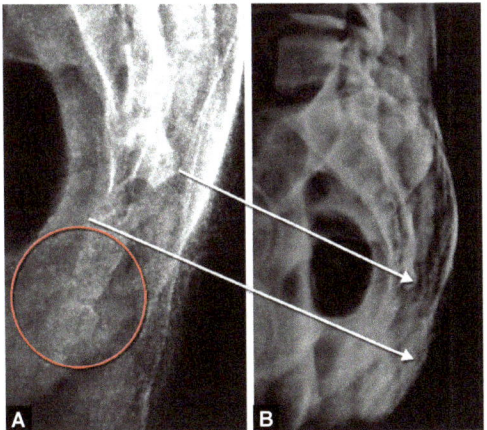

Figs. 4.13A and B: (A) Before surgery loose coccyx piece; (B) After surgery, it is excised.

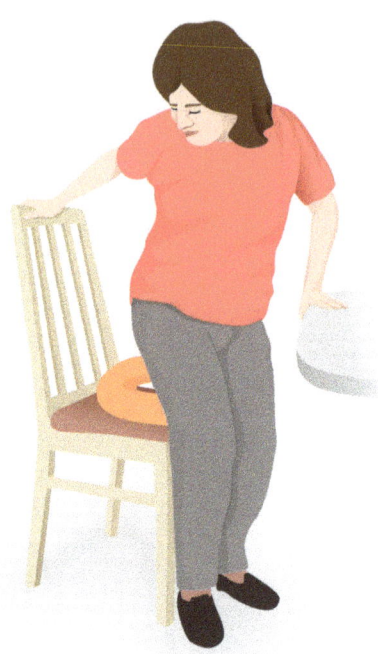

Fig. 4.14: Postoperative use cushion while sitting.

Burn every bleeding spot before closure. Subcutaneous tight closure is done, before skin closure. Water-tight dressing done, otherwise skin gets open out when patient is sitting. Use cushion while sitting. Induce constipation for 2 days. Skin closure with sutures, only after subcutaneous closure, so no skin tension. Water-tight dressing, otherwise skin gets open out when patient is sitting of wound. Use cushion while sitting (Fig. 4.14).

Chapter 5

Comminuted Fracture

DD Tanna

- Reamed (only in canal, bypassing the comminuted piece)
- Medullary cannel stuffing thick nail (to avoid early breakage)
- Static mode (never to dynamize)
- Secondary bone grafting (if needed)
- Maintaining the length (even if some fracture fragments in distraction) (Figs. 5.1 to 5.6).

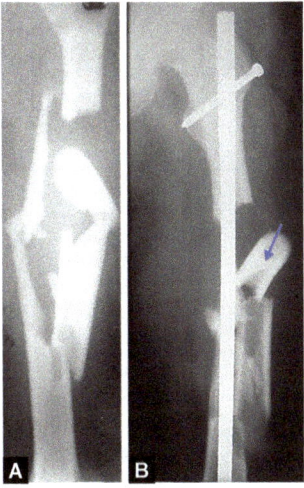

Figs. 5.1A and B: Closed nailing length maintained, nail threading of only major piece, rotated fragment (arrow).

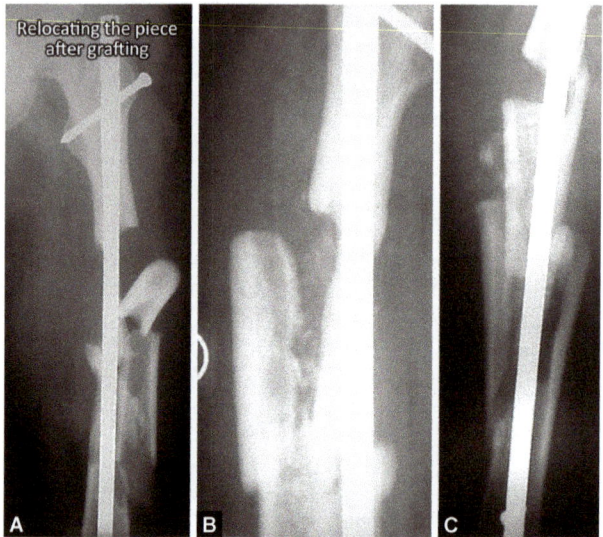

Figs. 5.2A to C: Nailed maintaining the length.

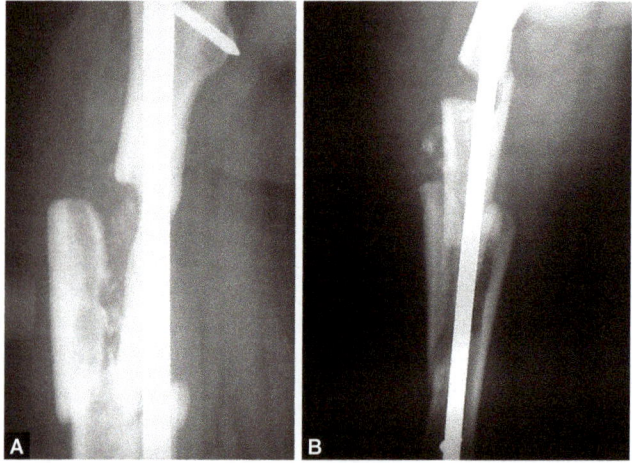

Figs. 5.3A and B: Relocating the piece and after grafting at a later date.

Chapter 5: Comminuted Fracture 43

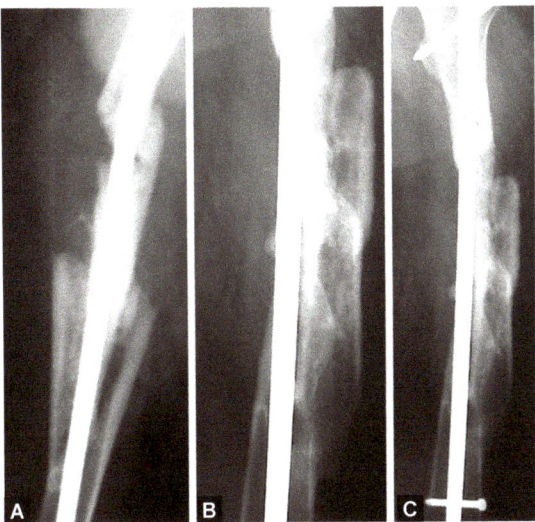

Figs. 5.4A to C: 18 months after grafting.

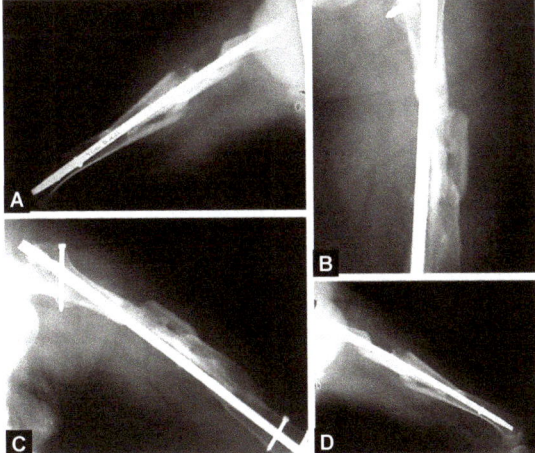

Figs. 5.5A to D: 24 months after grafting fracture healed without shortening and without any deformity.

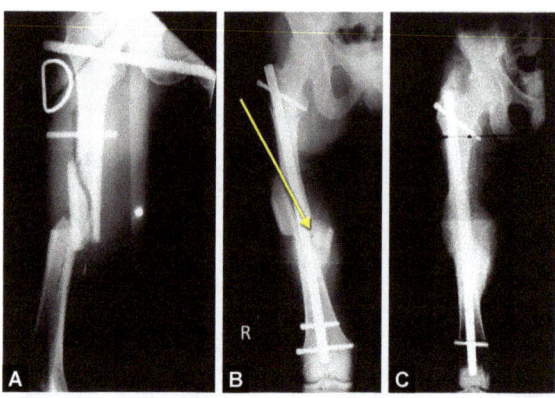

Figs. 5.6A to C: Comminuted fractures nailed with some distraction, which healed with no shortening and deformity.

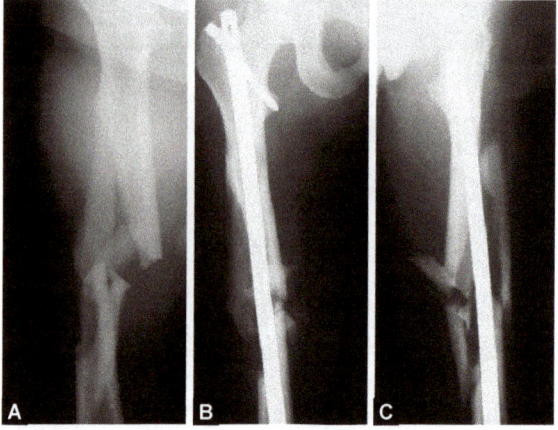

Figs. 5.7A to C: Comminuted fracture healed with nail in distraction, to maintain length.

Nail or plate is put in distraction, keeping normal length of the limb. Gap can be filled up latter in few weeks with an autograft or a segment transport (Figs. 5.7 and 5.8). It is better than lengthening with Elizarov (Figs. 5.9 to 5.12).

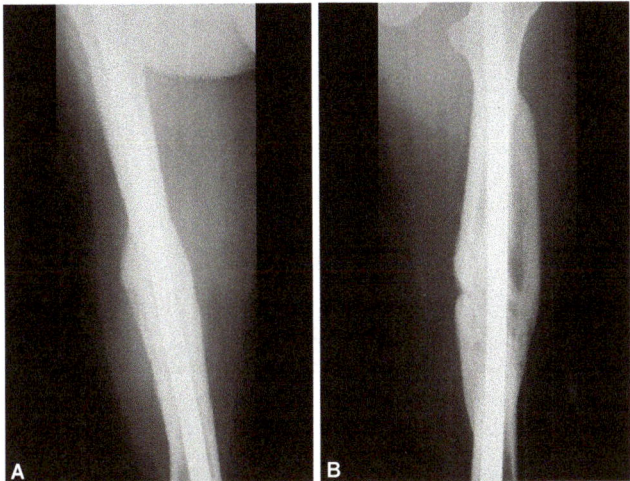

Figs. 5.8A and B: Observe that all segments are long oblique. Best healing potentials.

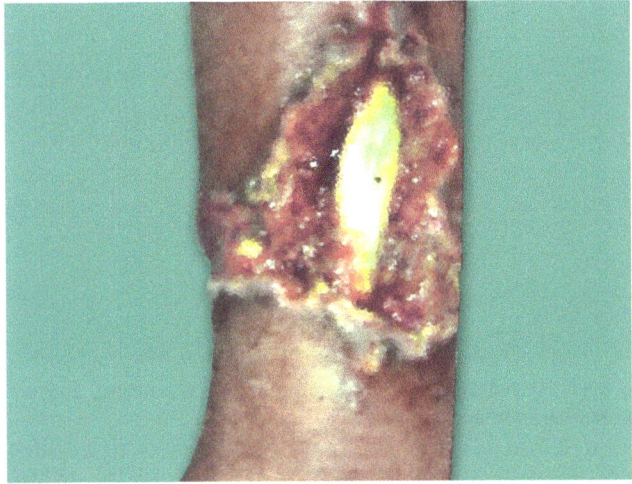

Fig. 5.9: Compound comminuted tibia.

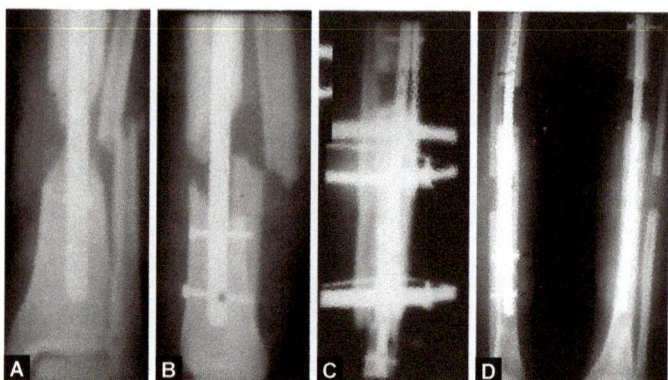

Figs. 5.10A to D: Nailed in distraction, once wounds heal segment, transport is done.

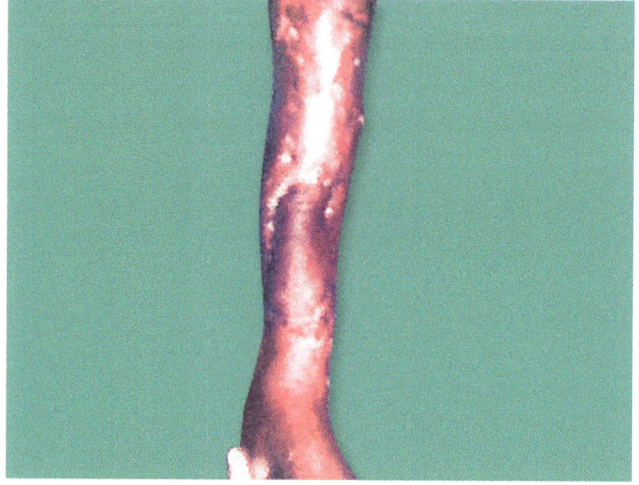

Fig. 5.11: Healed limb without deformity and shortening, and with segment transport and skin flap.

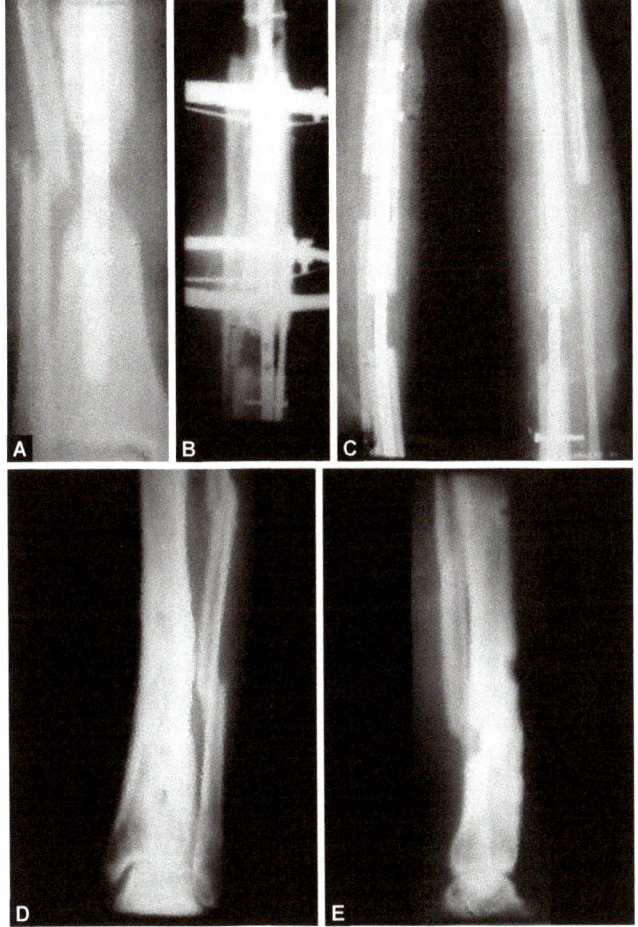

Figs. 5.12A to E: Final results.

Comminuted fracture is fixed in normal length and grafted after about 6 weeks (Figs. 5.13 to 5.18).

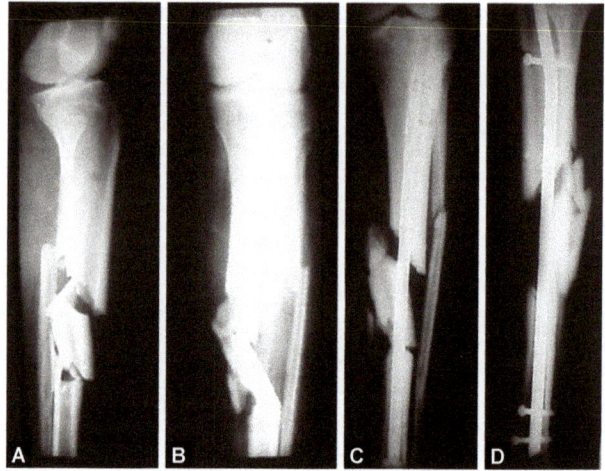

Figs. 5.13A and D: Comminuted fracture nailed with limb length equalized.

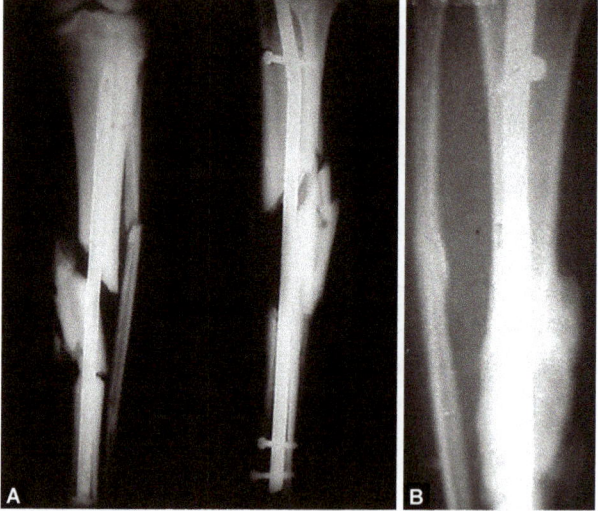

Figs. 5.14A and B: (A) Grafted; (B) Healed.

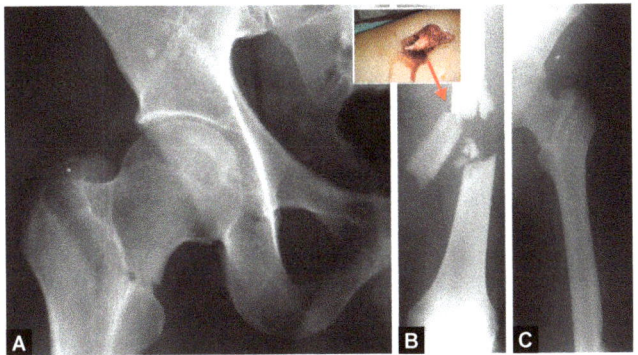

Figs. 5.15A to C: Comminuted fracture shaft femur with devitalized fragment of femur and ipsilateral neck femur fracture.
Courtesy: Dr RM Chandak, Nagpur.

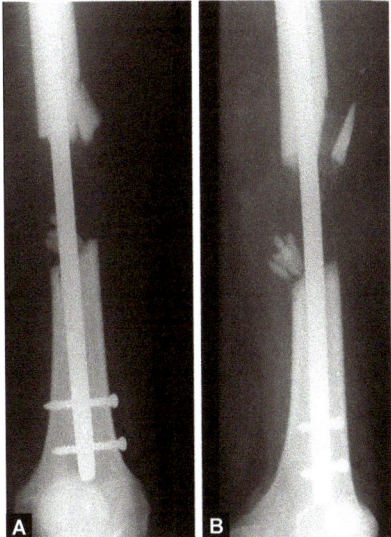

Figs. 5.16A and B: Postoperative check X-rays after interlock nailing, maintaining the length.

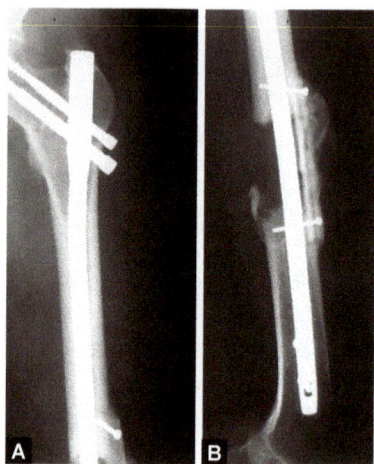

Figs. 5.17A and B: Fibula graft and auto cancellous graft for repair. Once wound is clean.

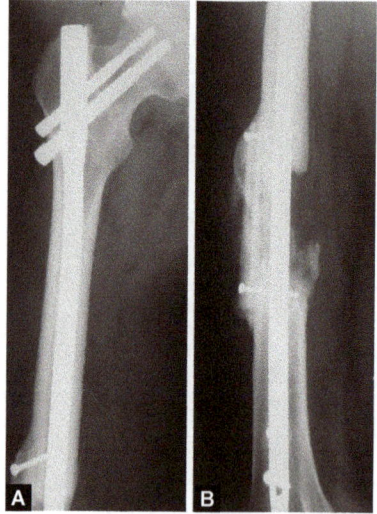

Figs. 5.18A and B

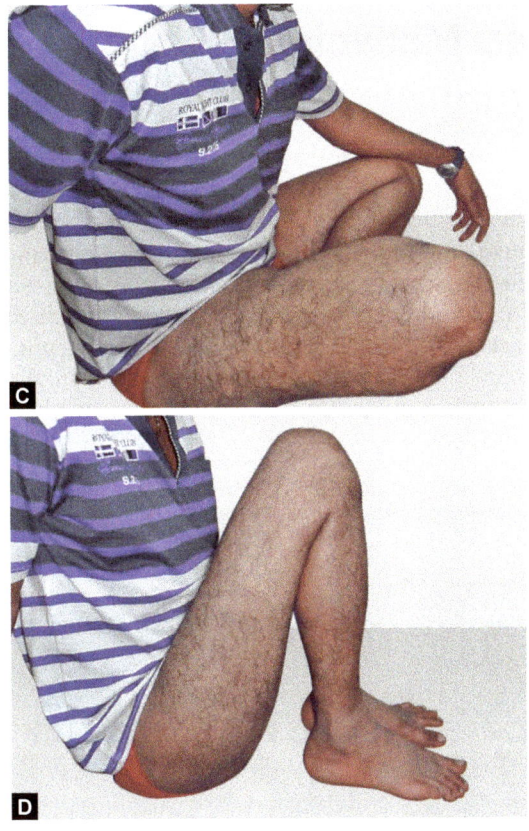

Figs. 5.18C and D

Figs. 5.18A to D: Fracture healed with full function.

Distal Transverse Medial Malleolus Fracture

Chapter 6

DD Tanna

Medial malleolus is treated with screw or tension band. This type of distal medial malleolus such as in Figure 6.1, needs a little extra attention. Such medial malleolus is suggested, first put wire vertical (arrow, Fig. 6.1) to the fracture, coming out on top of malleolus. Then put second or third wire and neutralize with tension band (Figs. 6.2 to 6.4). Only two oblique wires do not give stability (Fig. 6.5).

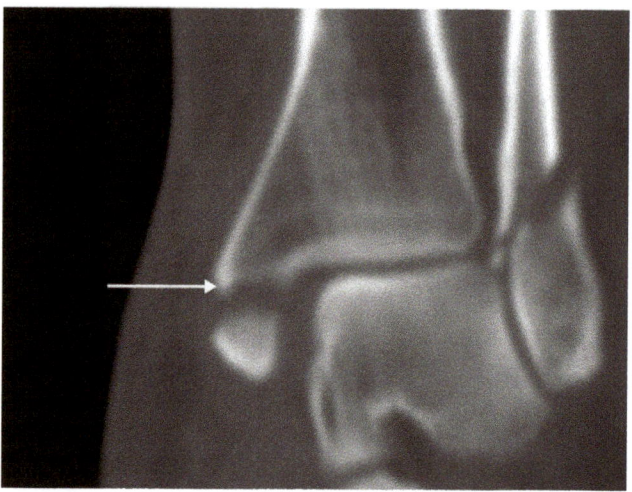

Fig. 6.1: Medial malleolus in distal; transverse fracture.

Chapter 6: Distal Transverse Medial Malleolus Fracture

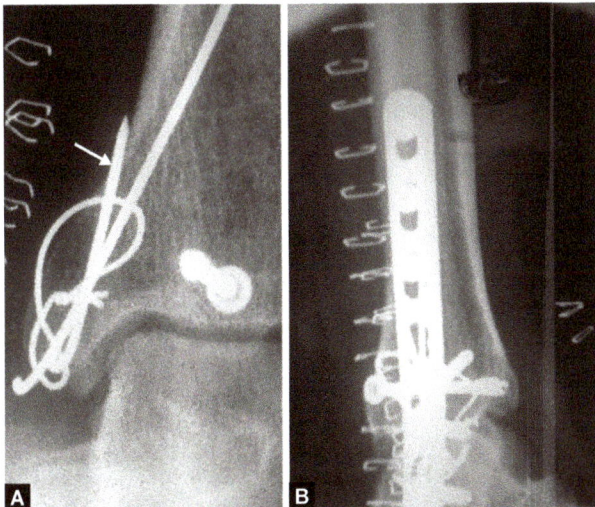

Figs. 6.2A and B: This type of distal fracture it is suggested, first put wire vertical (arrow) to the fracture, coming out on top of malleolus. Then put second or third wire and neutralize with tension band.

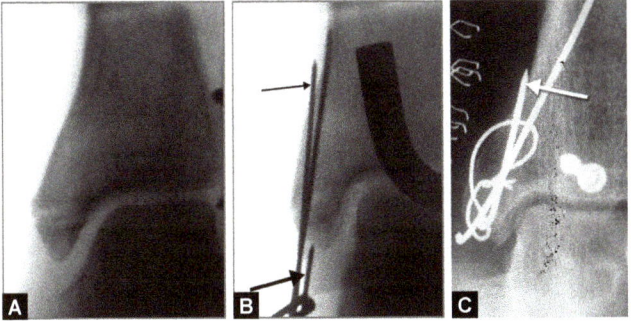

Figs. 6.3A to C: (A) Distal fracture; (B) It is fixed with tension band. K-wire (thin arrow) is passed first vertical to the fracture. Having transfixed, it can be improved with second wire (thick arrow); (C) After fixing this first wire perfectly (white arrow), other wires are passed and tension band is applied.

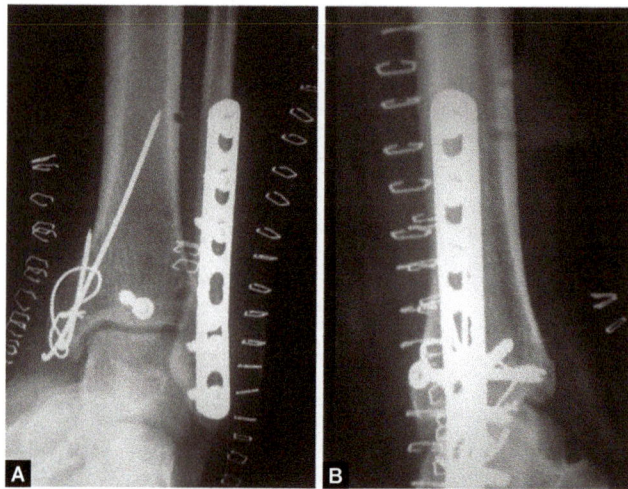

Figs. 6.4A and B: Final construct, medial malleolus fixed, and posterior. malleolus fixed with screw.

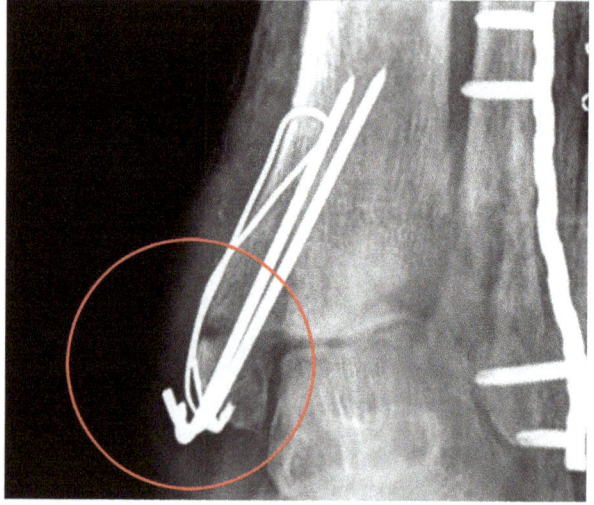

Fig. 6.5: Fracture can be mal-reduced, if reduction is not done by opening the joint.

Other suggestion, in order to achieve perfect reduction of all medial malleolus fracture, open capsule on medial malleolus and match distal end of tibia with medial malleolus perfectly before fixing (Figs. 6.6 and 6.7).

Case of malunited ankle, redone (Figs 6.8 and 6.9).

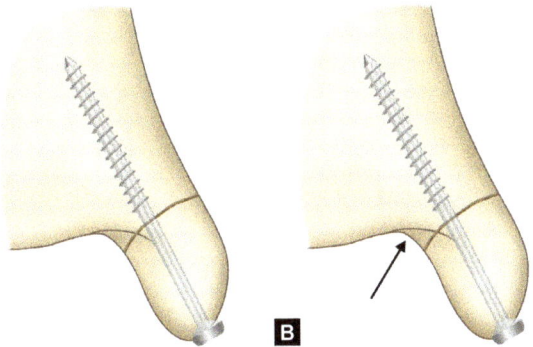

Figs. 6.6A and B: (A) While reducing medial malleolus, open the joint anteriorly and confirm perfect reduction; (B) Once capsule is opened, confirm the reduction by seeing relationship of distal tibia and medial malleolus. At times, there is rotation of this piece which needs to be corrected.

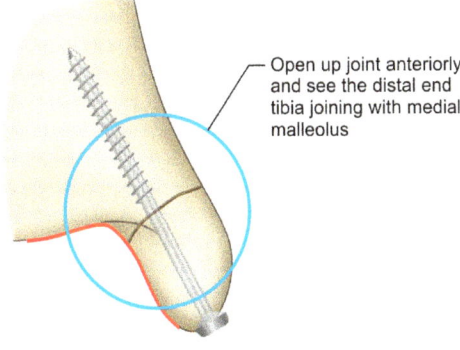

Open up joint anteriorly and see the distal end tibia joining with medial malleolus

Fig. 6.7A

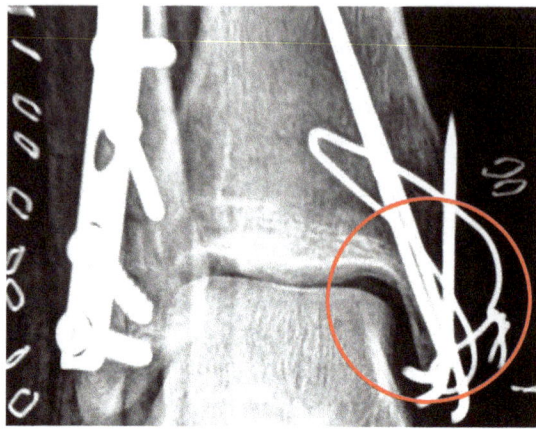

Fig. 6.7B
Figs. 6.7A and B: (A) Open capsule; (B) Observe perfect reduction of the medial malleolus.

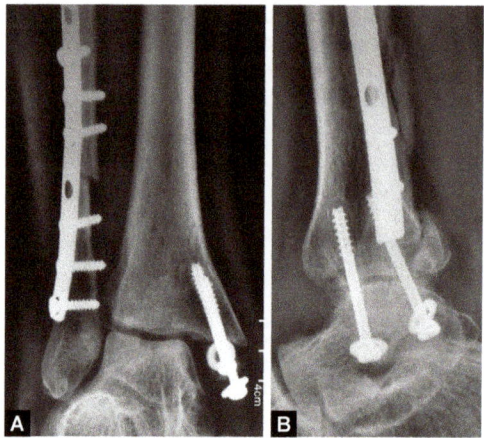

Figs. 6.8A and B: Patient came with this medial malleolus mal-reduced, and without fixation of posterior malleolus.

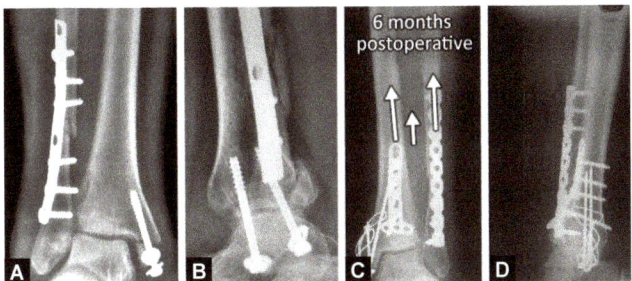

Figs. 6.9A to D: Low medial malleolus transverse fracture will not be fixed adequately with screw fixation. All these fragments must be anatomically fixed. When possible re-create what nature created, as it must have some specific function.

Head is Stronger than Machines (Investigations)

Chapter 7

DD Tanna

Here again we shall take patients and case scenarios to get the message home.

PROLAPSED INTERVERTEBRAL DISC

Patient presents with low back pain radiating to lower limb. On examination, straight leg raising (SLR) test is positive and neurological signs are also positive. MRI too shows a large disk (Figs. 7.1 and 7.2). Patient is advised surgery. He comes after 5 days to get admitted before day of surgery saying—"Sir there

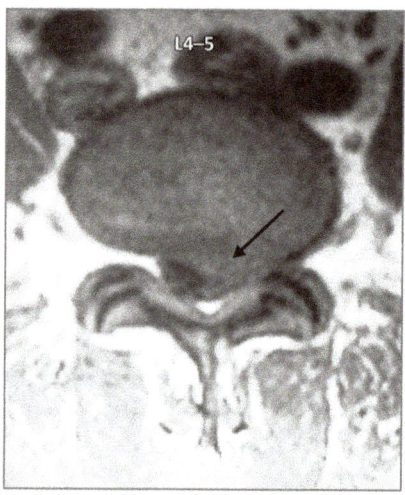

Fig. 7.1: Massive disk prolapse with sciatica.

Chapter 7: Head is Stronger than Machines (Investigations)

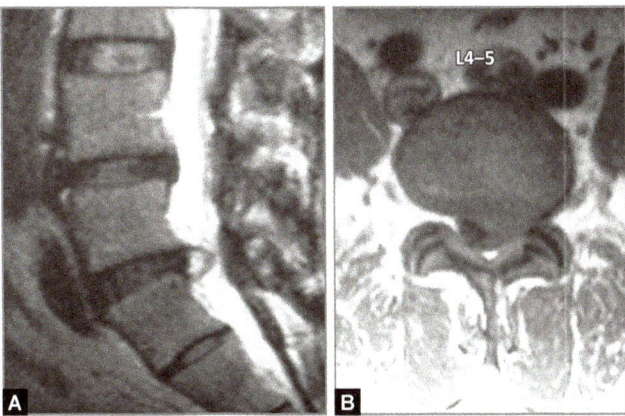

Figs. 7.2A and B: Massive disk prolapse.

is no pain in the leg or back, do I need surgery?" You examine the patient, SLR is normal and there are no positive findings. A repeat MRI shows same large disk. Now the advice is no surgery. Head has ruled over machine.

STERNOCLAVICULAR SWELLING

Patient usually presents with persistent swelling of the sternoclavicular joint as the main symptom (Fig. 7.3). Benign inflammation of this joint is seen with minimal symptoms without any deterioration over a long period of time. Investigations show a negative Mantoux test, CT/MRI show inflammation without obvious erosions or minor erosions (Figs. 7.4 to 7.6). Biopsy shows chronic inflammation. Trial of anti-TB drugs does not solve the problem. The swelling continues without any increase in pain, abscess or sinus formation even if it is not treated. If the swelling is minimally painful, stationary over a long period of time, leave it alone before going for biopsy. I am talking about only stationary non/minimally painful swelling. If swelling is increasing with pain—you must rule out other pathology.

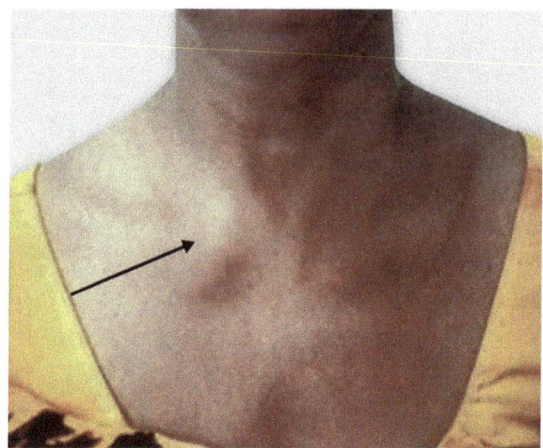

Fig. 7.3: Benign inflammation of sternoclavicular joint is seen with minimal symptoms without any deterioration over the period. Persistent sternoclavicular swelling is the main symptom.

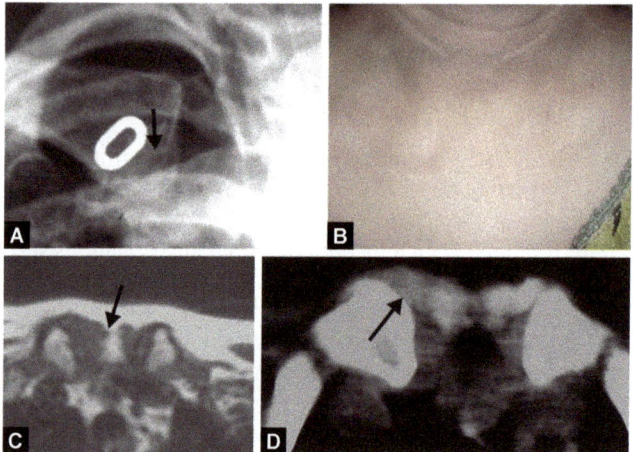

Figs. 7.4A to D: Negative Mantoux. CT/MRI show inflammation without obvious erosions or minor erosions. Biopsy shows chronic inflammation. Therapeutic trial of anti-TB drugs does not solve.

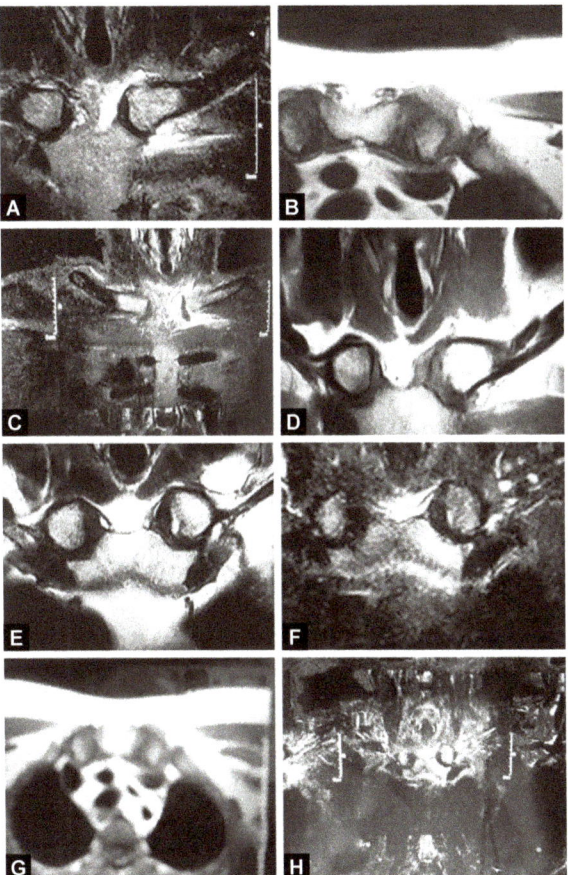

Figs. 7.5A to H: MRI images of sternoclavicular swelling. Leave it alone before going for biopsy in minimally painful, stationary swelling.

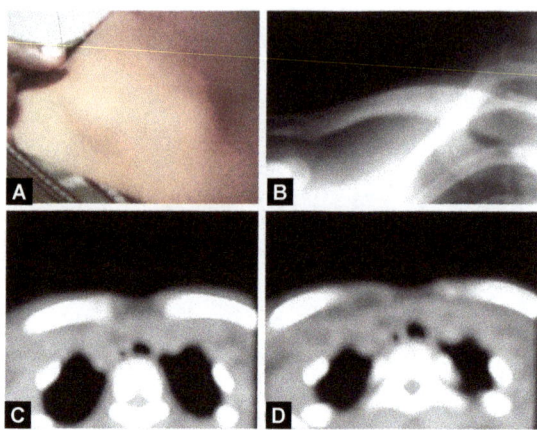

Figs. 7.6A to D: If increasing swelling with pain, must rule out other pathology. While advocating observation I am talking only about stationary, non painful swelling. Do not be in hurry to operate.

SYNOVIAL HERNIATION PIT OF FEMORAL NECK

A 30-year-old young male presents with complaints of pain in hip joint for months. On examination, movements are normal but pain on flexion and adduction. There is no localized tenderness or positive contributory history with normal X-ray reports. Despite analgesics and other means of conservative management, pain persists. MRI report too comes out to be normal, hence I asked for CT scan of hip as I felt MRI is not picking up the lesion. CT showed a localized circumscribed benign-looking lesion in the femoral neck (Figs. 7.7 and 7.8). Patient was operated, hip joint was approached anteriorly. The localized lesion was identified with C-arm help and curated out (Figs. 7.9 to 7.12). The curated material was sent for biopsy. The diagnosis was herniation (synovial) pit (Figs. 7.13 and 7.14). Synovial membrane goes in the bone and erodes the bone, making this benign impression on the bone. What is the reason of pain and why it gets cured by curettage is unexplained.

Chapter 7: Head is Stronger than Machines (Investigations)

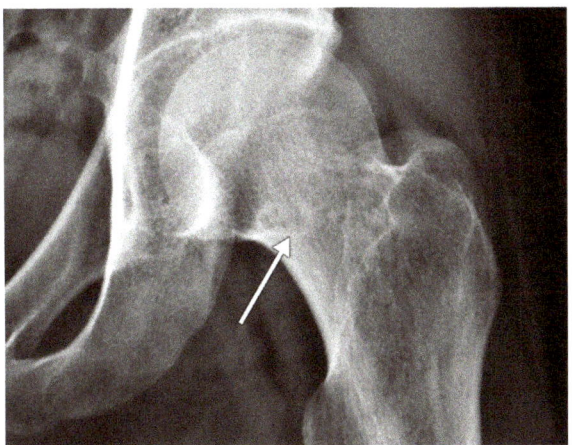

Fig. 7.7: A young man 35-year-old with pain in hip area for 2 years. X-ray shows lytic area.

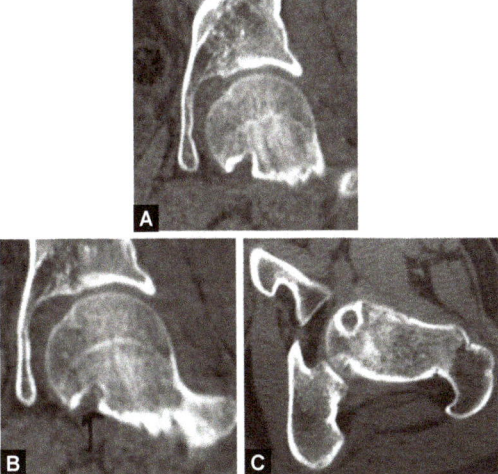

Figs. 7.8A to C: CT images show lytic lesion.

Orthopedic Secrets

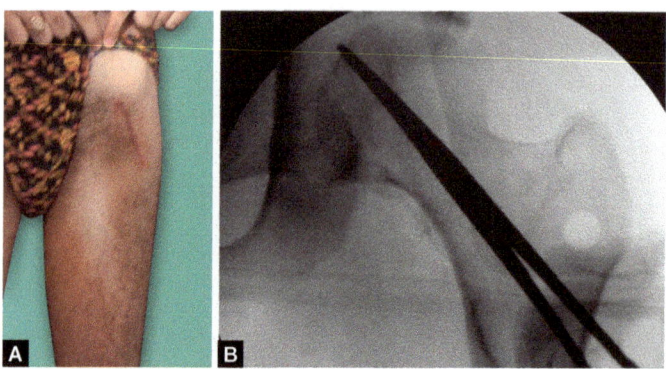

Figs. 7.9A and B: (A) Smith-Peterson approach anterior incision; (B) Lower party of neck lytic lesion localization.

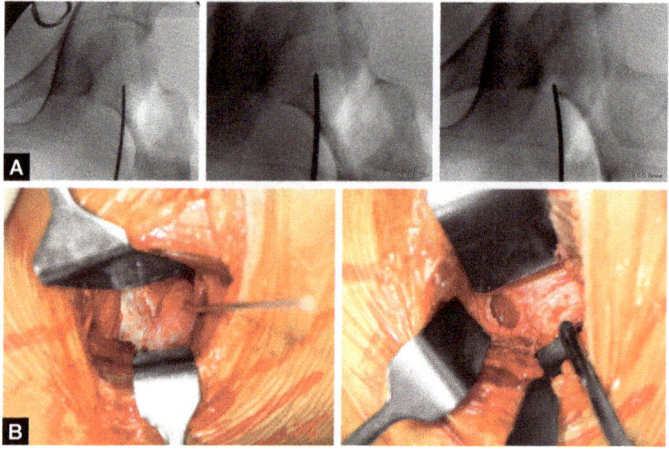

Figs. 7.10A and B: (A) Radiological localization; (B) Opening it after scraping, lytic lesion.

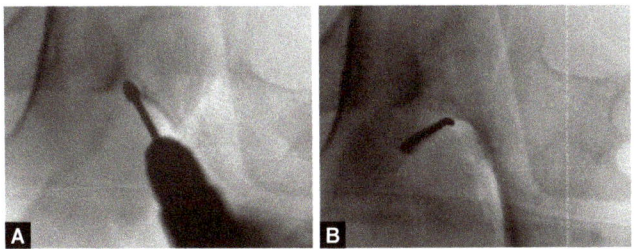

Figs. 7.11A and B: Scraping with high speed bur.

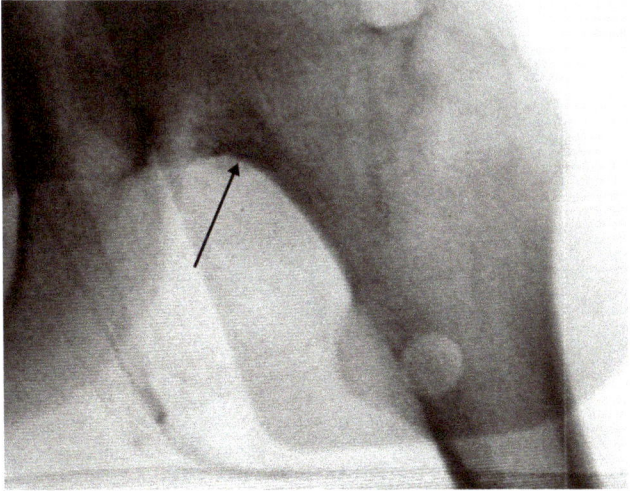

Fig. 7.12: Grafting.

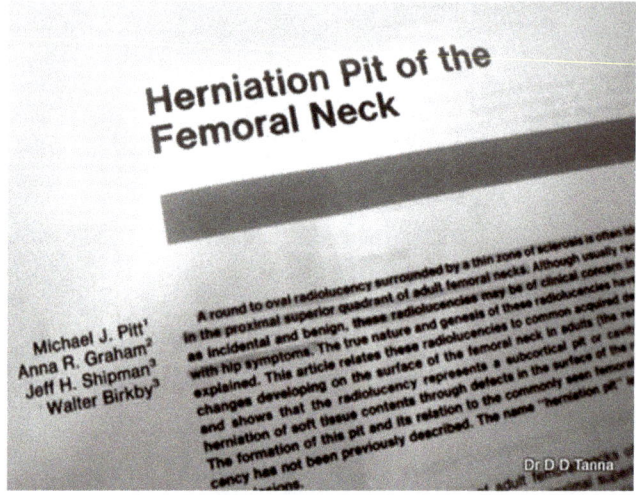

Fig. 7.13: Histology of curetted material shows herniation pit.

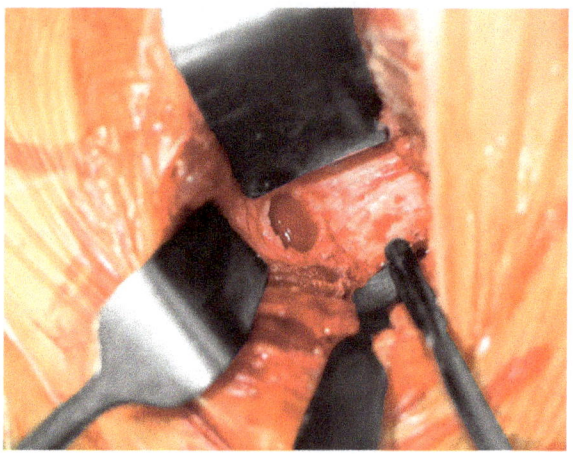

Fig. 7.14: Herniation (synovial) pit. Synovial membrane goes in the bone and erodes bone making this benign impression on the bone. Reason of pain here is unexplained.

ACETABULAR TUBERCULOSIS

A 40-year-old male was presented with complaints of hip pain for 2 months. He had difficulty in squatting, sitting crossed-legged. On examination, his flexion and external rotation were restricted, rest examination was noncontributory. X-ray reported two bony islands (Figs. 7.15 and 7.16) in femur neck and greater trochanter (GT) region. MRI report was normal (Figs. 7.17 and 7.18). I could not explain my clinical findings even though months had passed and pain was persisting. I ordered a CT scan of hip as I felt the findings needed to be explained. CT

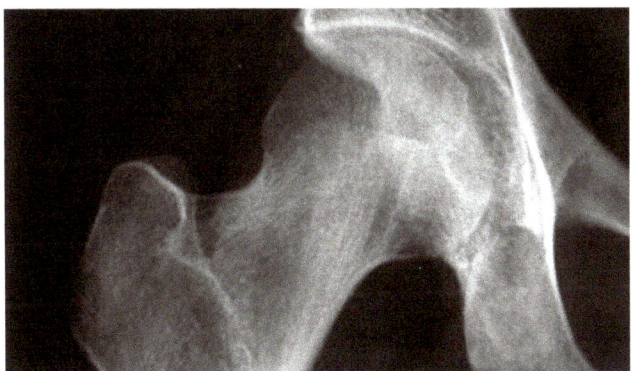

Fig. 7.15: X-ray normal.

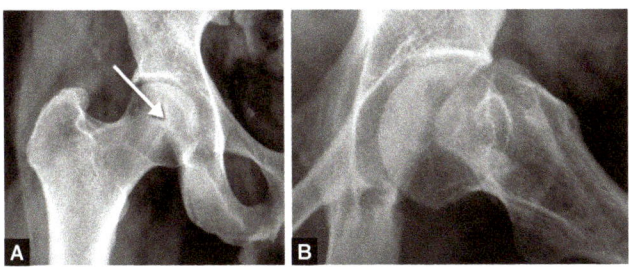

Figs. 7.16A and B: X-ray reported 2 islands, no significance.

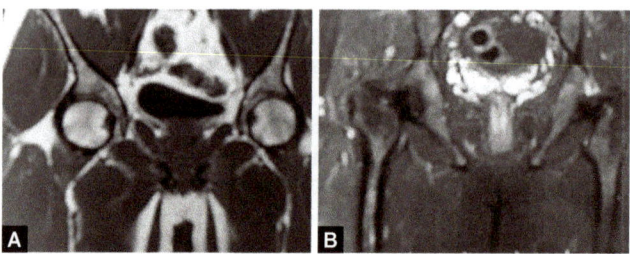

Figs. 7.17A and B: MRI normal.

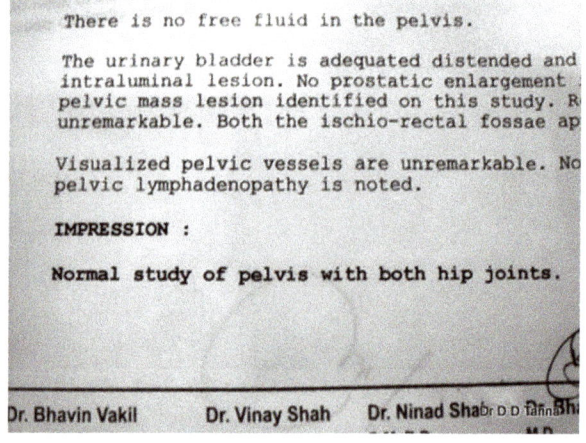

Fig. 7.18: MRI was reported as normal study.

showed lytic lesion in the posterior column of acetabulum (Fig. 7.19). The diagnosis was still not clear and the only way forward seemed a CT-guided biopsy. But I decided to give him trial of anti-TB drugs first. At the next follow-up, he was 40% better, movements had improved, and he had gained around 3 kg. I continued the AKT and patient recovered subsequently.

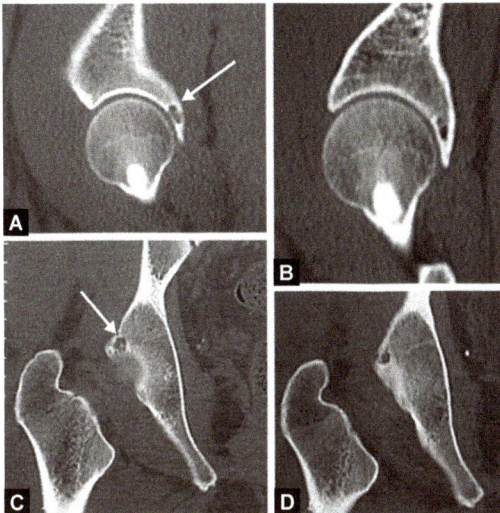

Figs. 7.19A to D: CT scan reveals lytic lesion in the posterior column of the acetabulum.

ENCHONDROMA OF FEMORAL HEAD

A 24-year-old male presented with minimal pain in hip. On examination, the hip was fully mobile, no restriction or deformity was found. MRI report brought by patient called it avascular necrosis (AVN) hip (Fig. 7.20). I was not convinced with this diagnosis as it did not fit with the findings of no deformity or loss of movement. Here I opted to get a CT-guided biopsy from a trusted place. CT was reported to be a cartilaginous neoplasm, possibly enchondroma. Now the treatment was clear. I went in through the anterior approach. Scooped out the pathological matter, burred the entire area with high speed bur, and the defect was bone grafted (Figs. 7.21 to 7.25).

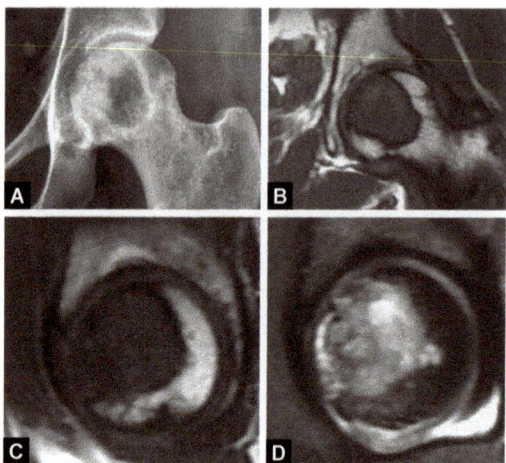

Figs. 7.20A to D: Reported outside Bombay as avascular necrosis (AVN), did not fit in my clinical observations. No deformity, no restriction. MRI localized lesion.

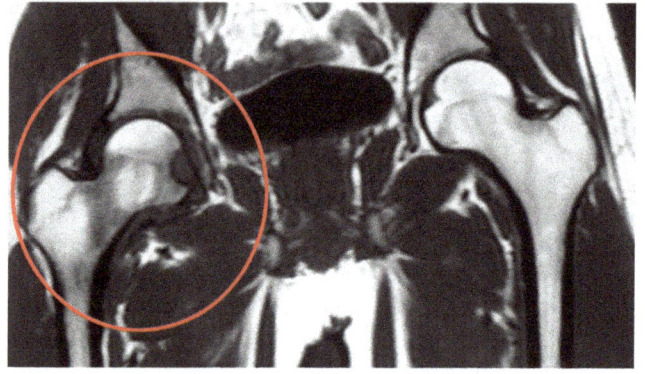

Fig. 7.21: A 20-year-old with minimal hip pain for 3 months. MRI image of the lesion.

Chapter 7: Head is Stronger than Machines (Investigations)

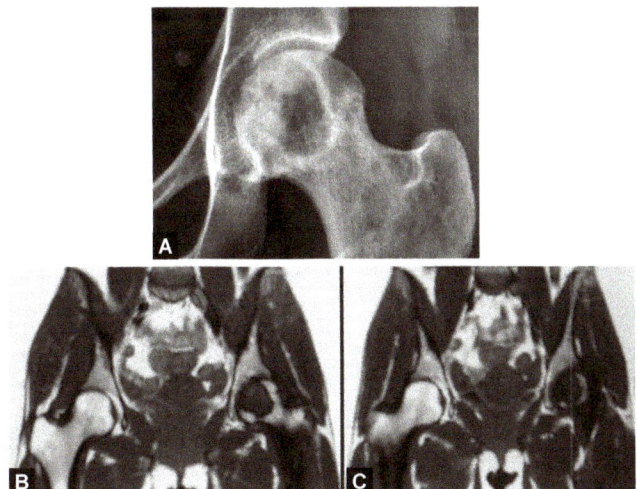

Figs. 7.22A to C: (A) X-ray; (B and C) MRI images of the lesion.

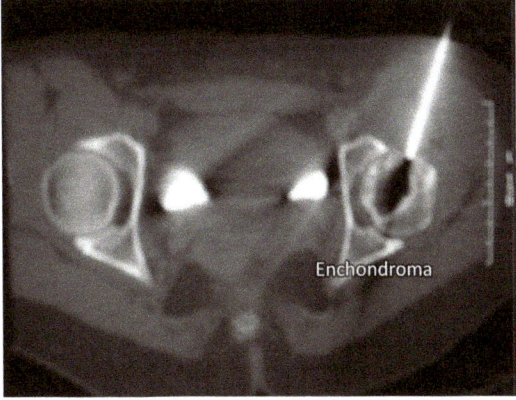

Fig. 7.23: CT guided biopsy done, histopath reported it to be enchondroma.

72 *Orthopedic Secrets*

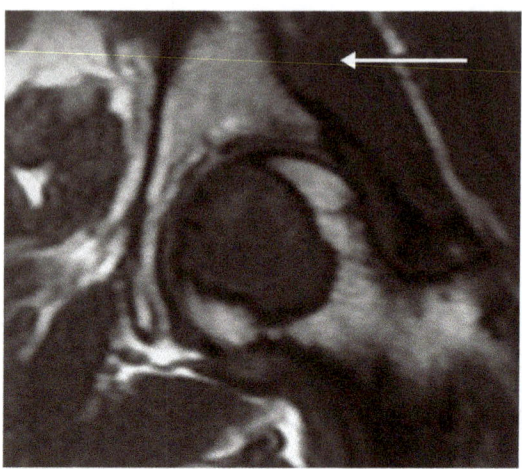

Fig. 7.24: MRI image of the lesion.

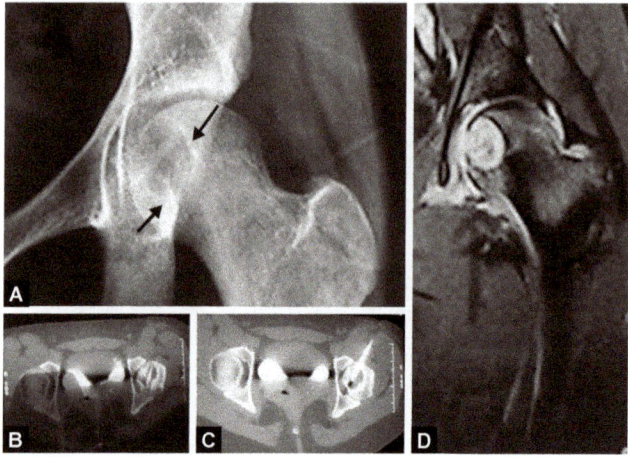

Figs. 7.25A to D: Grafted after curettage. (A) X-ray; (B to D) MRI images.

PAIN IN INGUINAL AREA

A 32-year-old young male was presented with pain and limp in right hip with difficulty in walking. Clinically, he had sharp tenderness in the inguinal region, restricted flexion and adduction with pain on flexion. MRI reported it to be effusion hip (Figs. 7.26 and 7.27); conservative symptomatic treatment did not give him relief. He had reached me after multiple consultations for elimination of hernia, varicosity in pelvis, and oncologist consultation—all of which were normal. About 5 months elapsed since onset of symptoms but the pain and inguinal tenderness persisted. On careful examination of the X-ray, I noticed a bony projection above the acetabulum (Figs. 7.28 to 7.31) not explained in the MRI report. I wrote a personalized note (Figs. 7.32 and 7.33) to the radiologist and requested him to dig up this matter for me. Fresh MRI and CT reports said it to be an overgrowth of

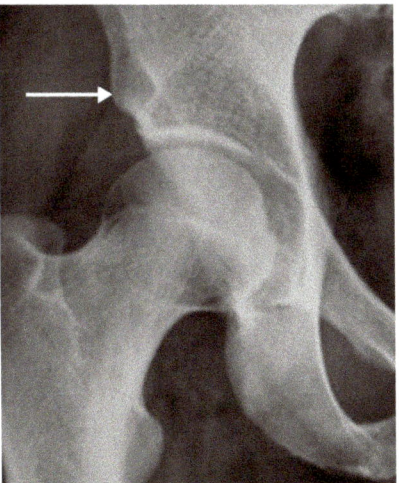

Fig. 7.26: A 32-year-old young male came with pain in right hip with positive findings of inguinal area tenderness. MRI reported effusion in hip. Symptomatic treatment gave no relief. This bony abnormality could not be explained.

74 *Orthopedic Secrets*

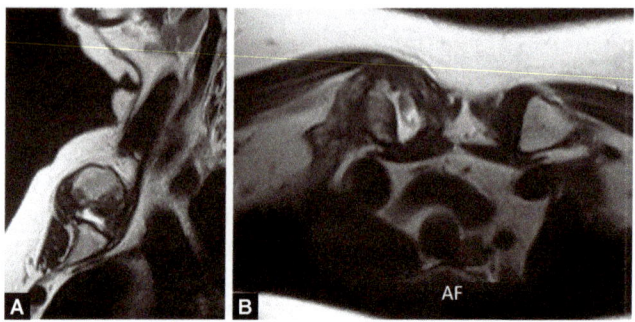

Figs. 7.27A and B: His MRI initially reported it to be effusion hip.

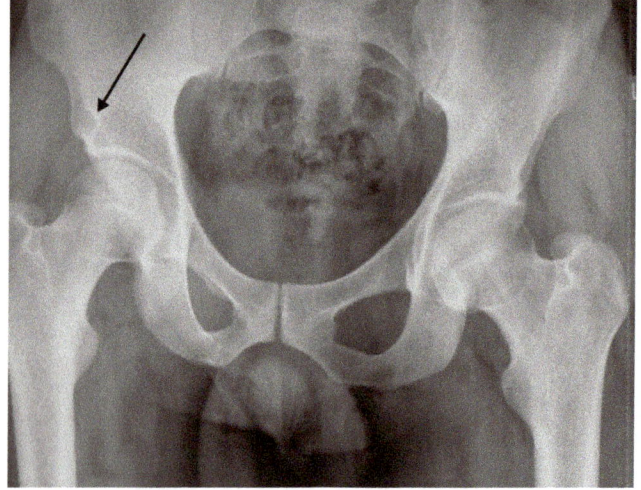

Fig. 7.28: Small bony projection (arrow) could not be explained.

Chapter 7: Head is Stronger than Machines (Investigations)

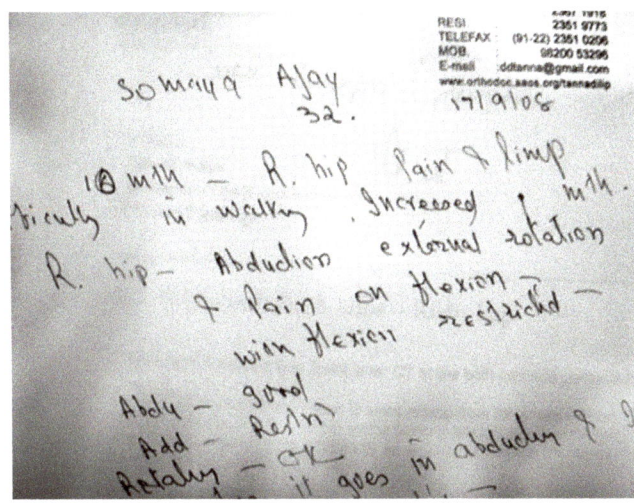

Fig. 7.29: My clinical notes during the first visit.

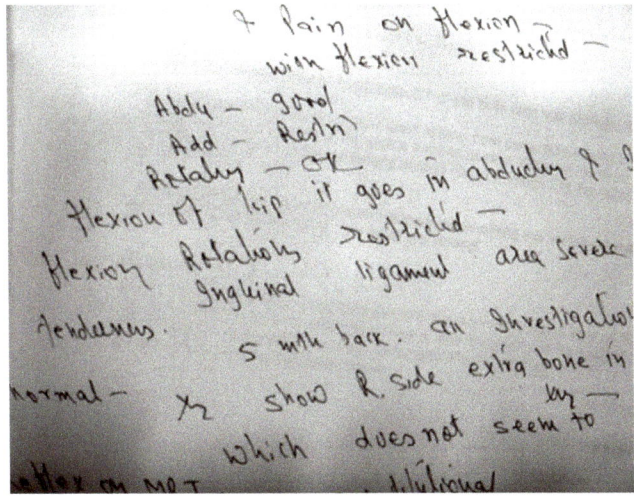

Fig. 7.30: Consultation notes.

Orthopedic Secrets

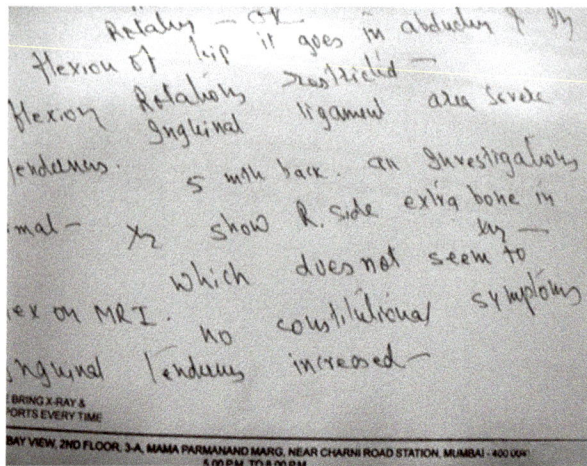

Fig. 7.31: My consultation notes.

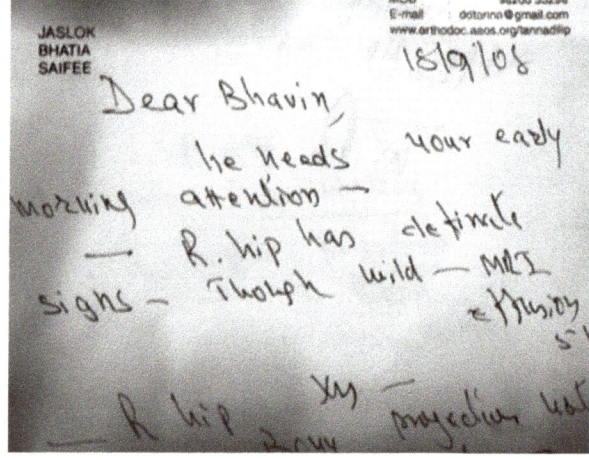

Fig. 7.32: My personal note to the radiologist.

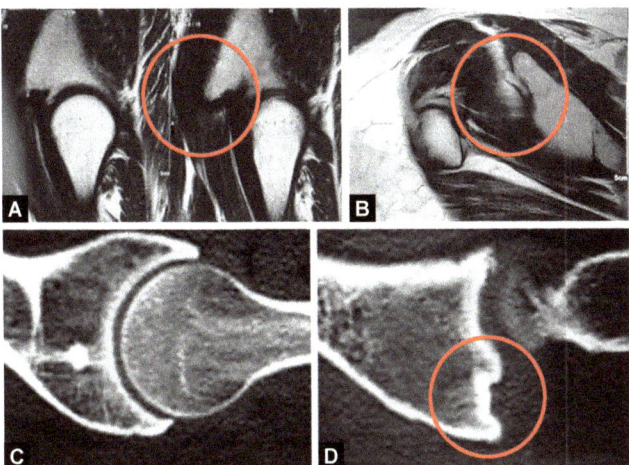

Figs. 7.33A to D: MRI image demonstrated it to be an overgrowth of bone at the origin of the rectus femoris tendon (anterior inferior iliac spine) suggestive of chronic avulsion sprain.

bone at the origin of the rectus femoris tendon (anterior inferior iliac spine) suggestive of chronic avulsion sprain (Fig. 7.34). Now we know what the issue was, local injection Depo-Medrol did the job (Fig. 7.35).

The point I am trying to make here is we all doctors are biased, we trust expansive investigations but not our God given free intellect. We all doctors miss many things at times. These are the few cases I picked up. There must be many I might have missed, someone else might have picked up. MRI report is not everything. As in the last case, my note to the radiologist hurt him and stimulated him to think. Clinical findings are and will always remain supreme. In the days of expansive investigations, we have forgotten clinical examination.

A plain high resolution and multiplanar CT of the both joint was performed

An unusual prolongation of bone is seen arising from the antero-inferior iliac spine, projecting along the origin of the rectus femoris tendon. Some of the tendon fibres arise from the bone a little more posteriorly as well (film 1 – image 21). No ossification is seen in this particular region.

A small osteophytes is seen postero-superiorly, involving the acetabular margin. The rest of the bones are normal. The joints are normal.

Remarks:
Correlating with the MRI, it appears that there is an overgrowth of bone at the origin of the rectus femoris tendon, with altered signal and irregularity at the origin of the tendon slips a little more posteriorly as well, all suggestive of a chronic avulsion sprain. The rest of the features are as described above.

is an overgrowth of bone at the or
and irregularity at the origin of the
stive of a chronic avulsion sprain.

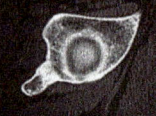

Fig. 7.34: MRI report from the radiologist.

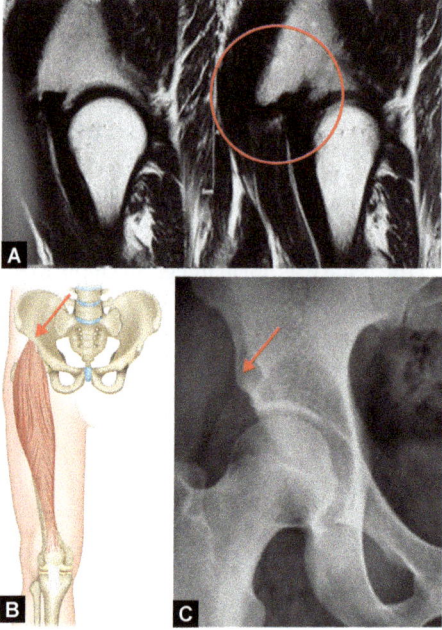

Figs. 7.35A to C: Local Depo-Medrol injection cured him. Now I know what is cause of pain.

POST-PREGNANCY PAIN IN BOTH HIPS

A 28-year-old post-pregnancy pain in both hips and inability to walk. Some pain had started during 5th month of pregnancy (Figs. 7.36 to 7.38).

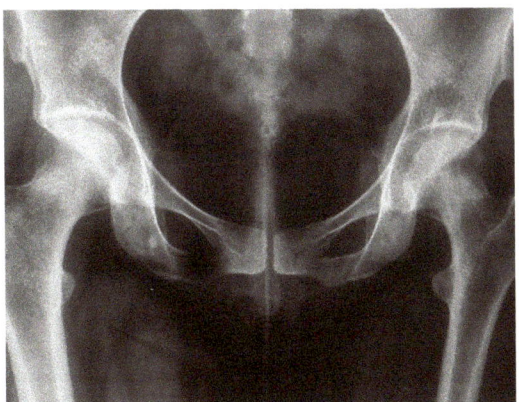

Fig. 7.36: A 28-year-old woman with post-pregnancy pain in both hips and inability to walk. Some pain had started during 5th month of pregnancy.

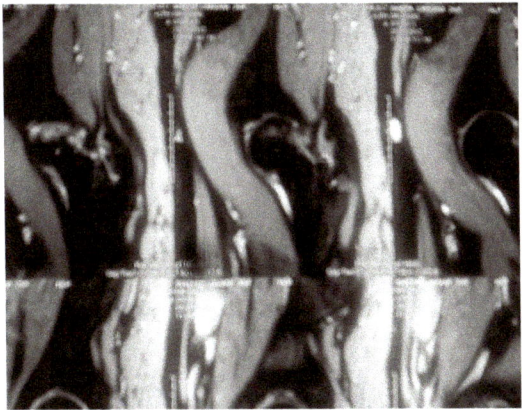

Fig. 7.37: MRI reported it as avascular necrosis (AVN) hips.

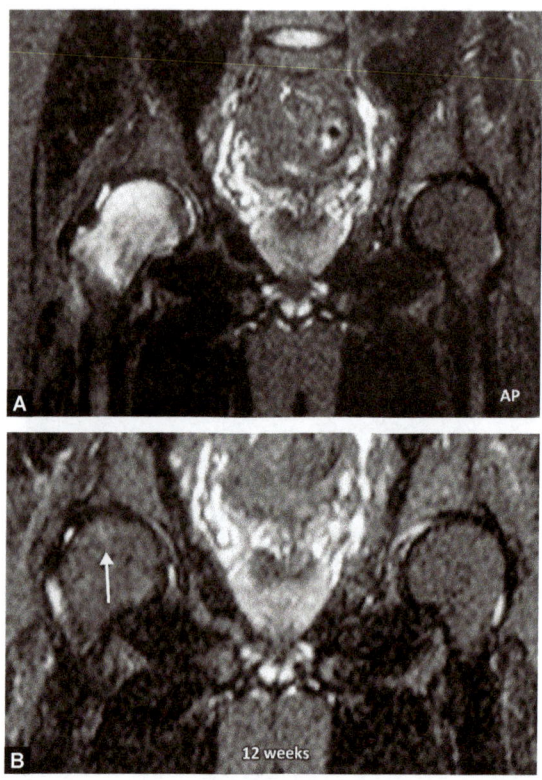

Figs. 7.38A and B: (A) Typical changes of idiopathic osteoporosis; (B) All changes disappear in 8–12 weeks time.

MRI was reported as AVN and patient was advised core decompression, my head did not agree with this report. I asked for review of the MRI images (Figs. 7.39 to 7.41). MRI was then reported as idiopathic osteoporosis, which is now also termed as insufficiency fracture. She was treated conservatively with vitamin D and calcium supplements. All changes were reversed and patient was saved from surgery.

Chapter 7: Head is Stronger than Machines (Investigations)

> rticular margins of both SI joints are normal without evidence of erosions. The
> ondral marrow of the sacro-iliac joints appears normal bilaterally. The joint space is
> reserved.
>
> of the bones reveal normal marrow signal.
>
> terus appears bulky with hemorrhagic fluid in the endometrial cavity consistent with
> artum status. Rest of the intrapelvic soft tissues structures are normal.
>
> **usion:**
>
> **: imaging features are suggestive of avascular necrosis of both femoral heads wi**
> **ve hip joint effusion. Marrow edema is seen in the femoral head and neck**
> **rally.**

Fig. 7.39: Original MRI report from the radiologist.

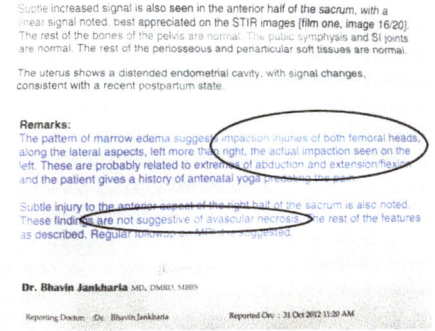

Fig. 7.40: Review MRI report.

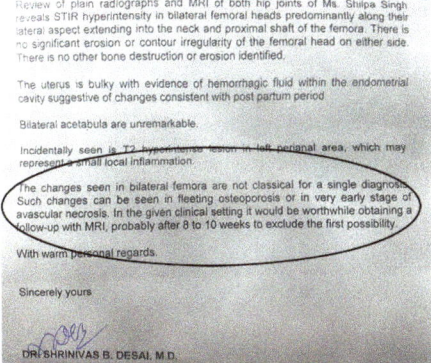

Fig. 7.41: Review MRI report by another independent radiologist.

PAIN IN HIP UNEXPLAINED

A 55-year-old healthy man was presented with pain in right hip for 4 weeks. Movements were almost full, with no deformity. 1st MRI showed nonspecific bone erosions (Fig. 7.42) and patient was advised biopsy. I was consulted for 2nd opinion. Clinically, he was almost normal, I was not convinced with the MRI. MRI signal changes, I decided to wait and watch. 2nd MRI was done at 3 weeks and I was surprised (Fig. 7.43). No radiologist agreed. Since changes had reduced, I held on. He improved. Last MRI report was normal (Fig. 7.44).

INFECTION AFTER 15 YEARS

A 50-year-old man was operated 15 years back and all was fine. He developed gradual onset of pain in operated part with warm, reddish, and painful skin. Osteomyelitis was diagnosed and treated. When I saw him, I observed patient was in pain but fully functional. X-ray was typical of metal reaction and not infection

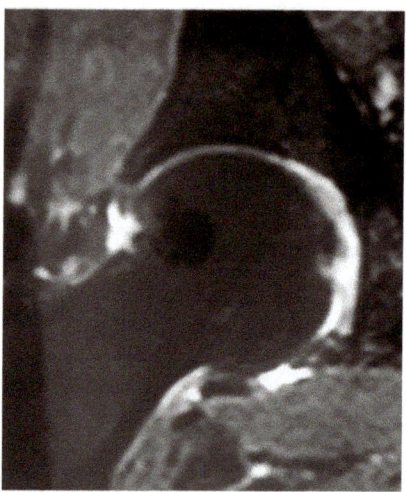

Fig. 7.42: A 55-year-old, pain in right hip for 4 weeks, came this MRI. 1st MRI showed nonspecific bony erosion.

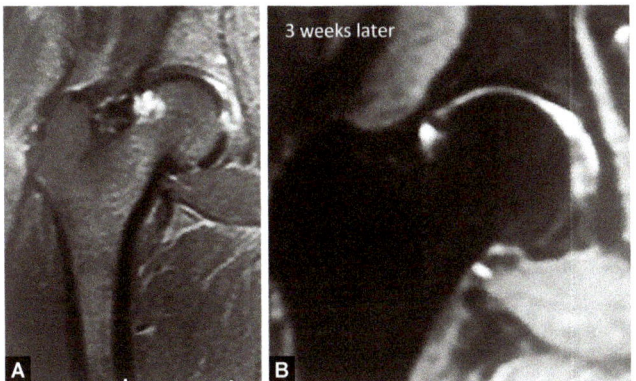

Figs. 7.43A and B: MRI at 3 weeks interval shows reduced signals.

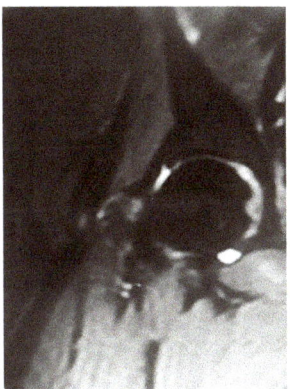

Fig. 7.44: Last MRI all clear.

(Fig. 7.45). This lysis is typical of metal reaction as seen by me in past. So patient was taken up for implant removal. As soon as I opened, black metallic debris came out. Broken end of the nail was seen all engulfed with this debris. Lytic area scraped and scooped out, and was filled with $CaSO_4$ with antibiotics (Figs. 7.46 to 7.49). Remaining nail could not be removed and patient had no problem for 2 years of follow-up.

Orthopedic Secrets

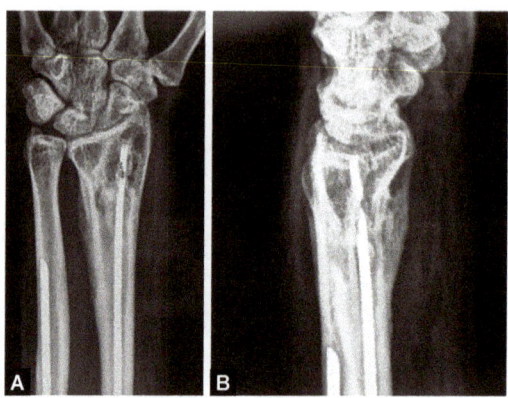

Figs. 7.45A and B: (A) Operated 15 years back, square nail *in situ*; (B) X-ray reported it as infection.

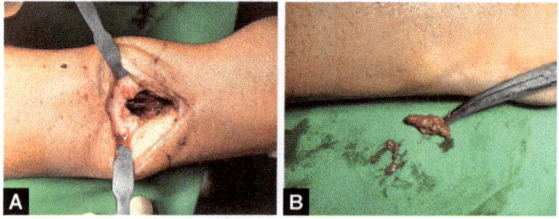

Figs. 7.46A and B: Black metallic debris.

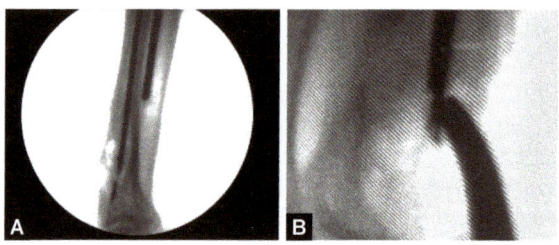

Figs. 7.47A and B: Broken square nail.

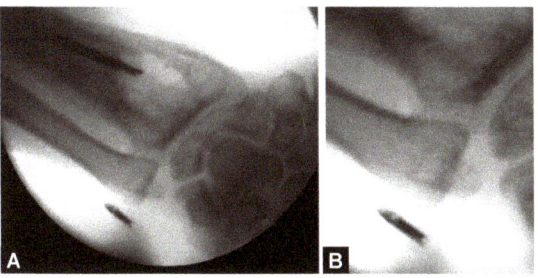

Figs. 7.48A and B: C-arm image after scraping and scooping out the debris. Broken part of nail was embedded in bone and could not be removed.

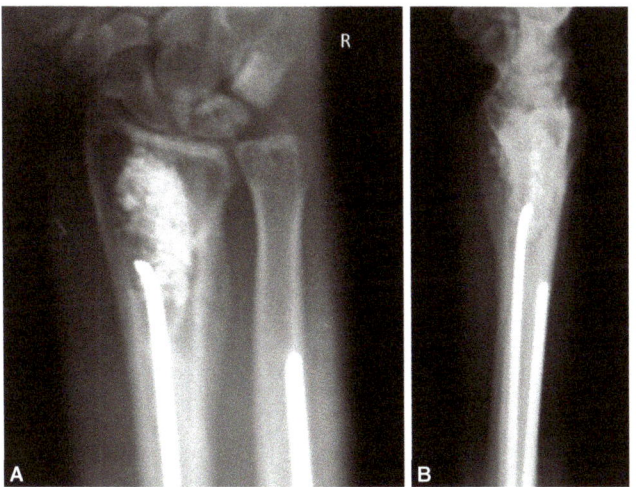

Figs. 7.49A and B: Lytic area scraped, and scooped out, and filled with $CaSO_4$ with antibiotics.

CONCLUSION

These days, with mushrooming MRI centers, reports of all are not dependable. We must correlate with our clinical examination whether the report fits.

Chapter 8

Implant Removal

DD Tanna

AUSTIN MOORE REMOVAL

Austin Moore prosthesis needs to be removed if required, particularly due to osteoarthritis of acetabulum only after 7–8 years of primary surgery (Figs. 8.1A to C) or if the prosthesis becomes loose immediately in 1 or 2 months' time after surgery (Figs. 8.2A and B). When it needs to be removed, if it is to be removed immediately, it is easier. After long time, it is not that easy.

Way to go about is (Fig. 8.3):
- Big thick capsule (pseudocapsule) is formed around the head of femur; it is not like normal capsule. It is like an hourglass hugging the metal all the time. This needs to be removed first.

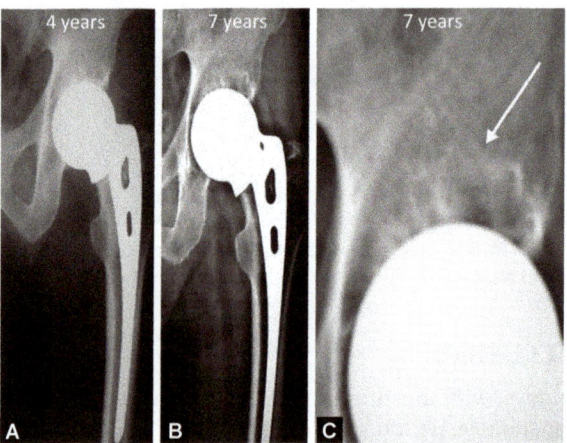

Figs. 8.1A to C: Arthritic changes in the acetabulum. (A) 4 years; (B) 7 years; (C) 7 years with arthritic changes in the acetabulum.

Chapter 8: Implant Removal

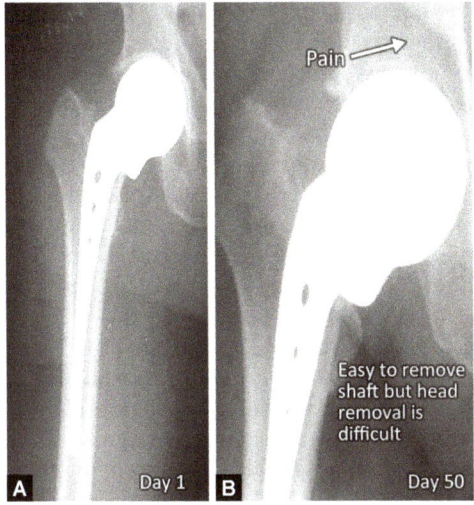

Figs. 8.2A and B: Loose prosthesis, needing early removal. (A) Day 1; (B) Day 50 with osteolysis indicating loose prosthesis.

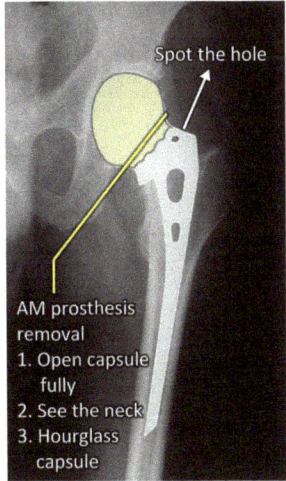

Fig. 8.3: Capsulectomy and not capsulotomy is needed for removal.

- Then after that we need to find the top hole of Austin Moore prosthesis on neck which is often covered by bone. Remove that bone and put bone hook in the top hole. After bone hook is placed, you have control over the prosthesis.

  With the help of hook, pull the head out little to the brim of acetabulum, and adduct the leg while doing this. Do not external rotate or internal rotate to dislocate before this. Once head is at the brim of acetabulum, it can be rotated to dislocate. Many times there is no space in the neck to enter for removal of bone from top holes (Fig. 8.4). We should always go from trochanter area on all sides except medially which is difficult. Clear the top of the prosthesis which is in trochanter. Remove bone with gouge and get prosthesis clear at the proximal part from trochanter (Fig. 8.5). Rarely, a trochanteric osteotomy is needed to remove this bone and prosthesis. Sometimes there is bone formation in the distal hole too (Figs. 8.6A and B).

  If the bone is formed in the hole distally, then we have to remove bone by breaking it *via* a guidewire directed at the

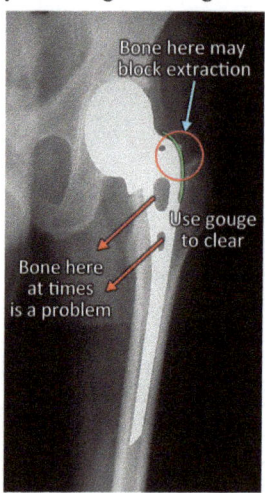

Fig. 8.4: Bone near the top hole requires removal with a bone gouge.

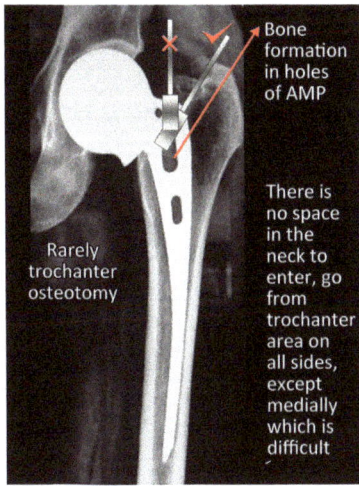

Fig. 8.5: Removal of bone may rarely need a trochanteric osteotomy.

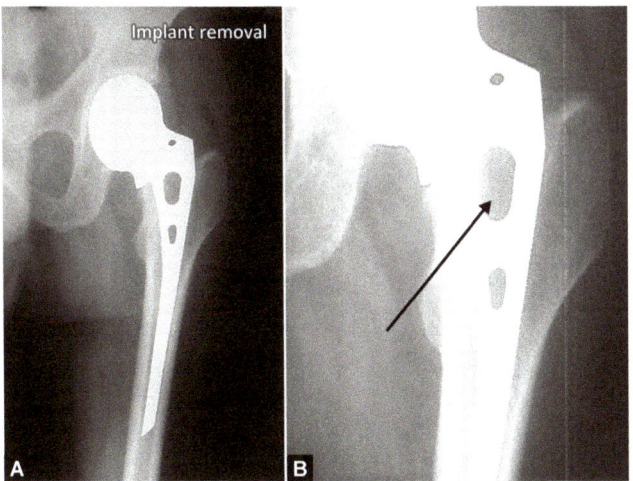

Figs. 8.6A and B: Bony ingrowth in the hole in the proximal stem of the prosthesis.

bone in the hole and drilling with cannulated drill bits like we do in interlocking (Figs. 8.7 to 8.11). Once bone is broken, prosthesis can be removed easily.

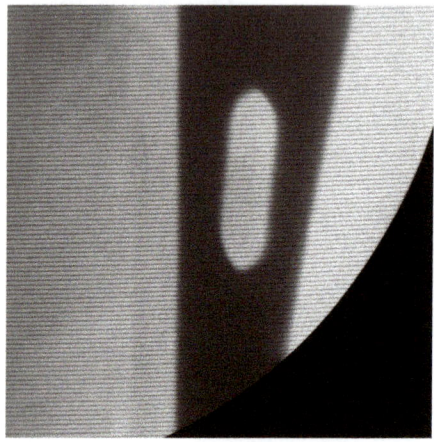

Fig. 8.7: Bone ingrowth in stem hole of prosthesis as seen in C-arm image.

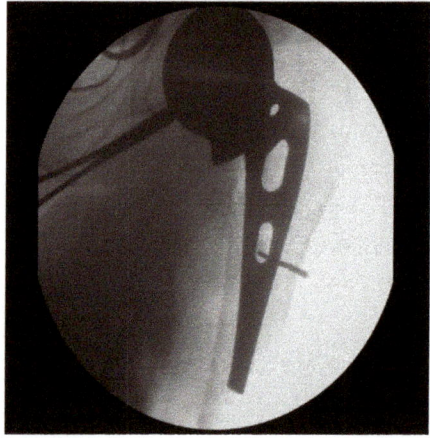

Fig. 8.8: Breaking the bony ingrowth with guidewire and cannulated drill bits.

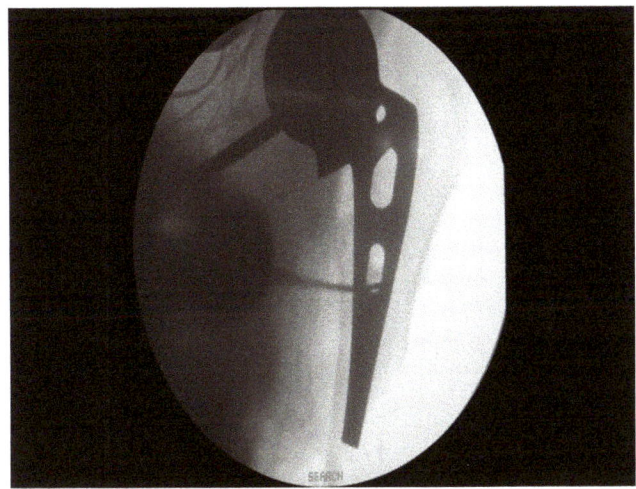

Fig. 8.9: Guidewire directed at the bone in the hole under C-arm guidance.

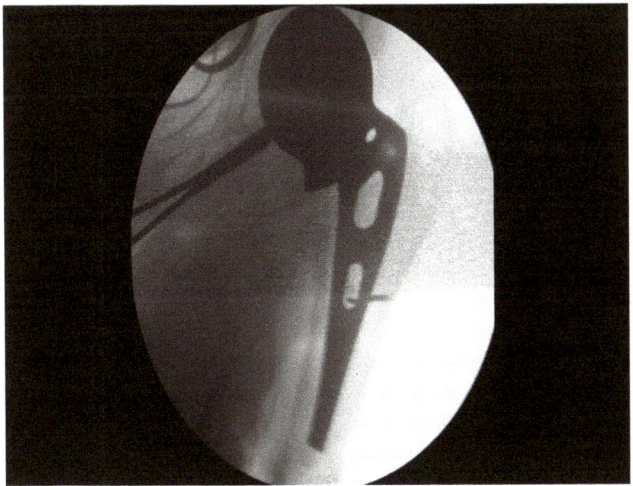

Fig. 8.10: Multiple drill holes might be needed to remove the entire bone block.

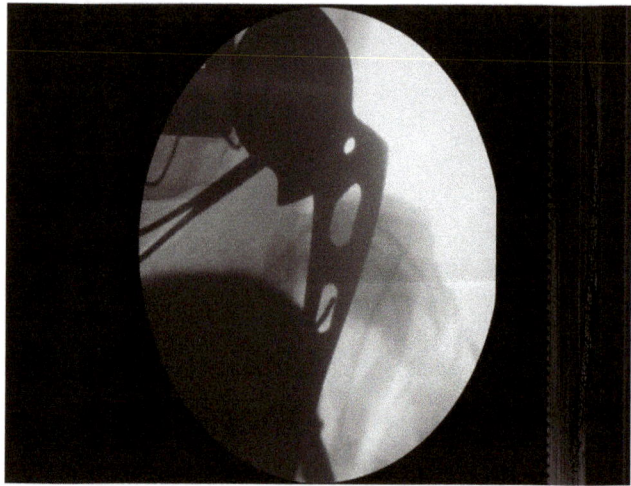

Fig. 8.11: Bone inside the hole being broken with cannulated drills.

In summary:
- Capsulectomy and not capsulotomy
- Do not use rotation of limb for removal.

DYNAMIC HIP SCREW REMOVAL

In dynamic hip screw (DHS) removal, the neck screw removal is the challenging part. DHS removal is needed mostly when the implant is broken or failed (cut through) or in infected cases.

If infected, then there is no issue in removing the DHS screw as it becomes loose and easily removable. But in noninfected cases, it is really difficult to remove as in most of the Indian implants, reverse cutting threads are not present. The way to go about is to use a hollow mill developed by myself which goes around the Richard screw. The bone around it is over drilled and then the screw is easily removed. Figures 8.12 and 8.13 show

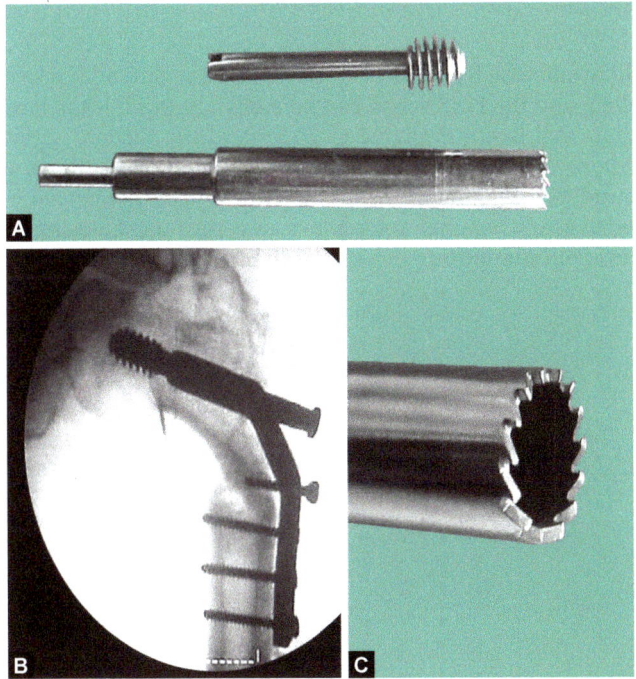

Figs. 8.12A to C: (A) Richard screw and special hollow mill for the large diameter; (B) Nonunion IT fracture with implant failure; (C) Large diameter special hollow mill.

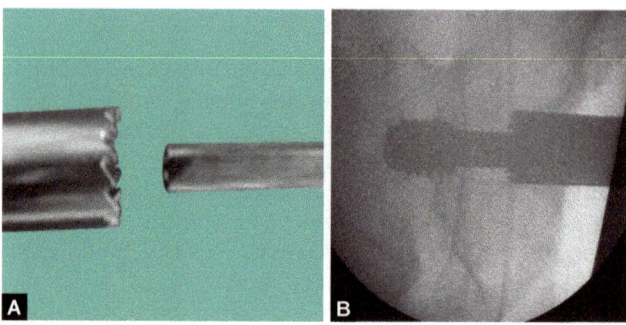

Figs. 8.13A (*In vitro*) and B (Intraoperative): Hollow mill removes bone blocking the Richard screw from coming out.

hollow mill which goes over screw head, bone around it is over drilled, and the DHS screw can be easily removed. If the large hollow mill is not available to go around the Richard screw, the bone around it should be broken with multiple drillings all around its circumference. Additionally, a bone gouge can be used to gently hammer and remove away the bone blocking the screw from coming out.

HUMERUS PLATE REMOVAL

Humerus plate is not necessary to be removed unless in cases of nonunion where patient needs revision surgery or associated infection. According to literature, incidences of radial nerve palsy are higher during plate removal as compared while doing primary surgery for fracture. Removal of plate is tricky in humerus as two heads of triceps are not separate during a second surgery and difficult to recognize. Sometimes they may have been stitched together during the primary surgery. So the trick is to go higher up under the deltoid and trace the radial nerve from virgin area on the medial side before traversing to lateral side as shown in the Figure 8.14.

To approach the screws, go directly through the muscles above the screw, clear the muscle with artery and remove it. There is no need to cut the whole muscle.

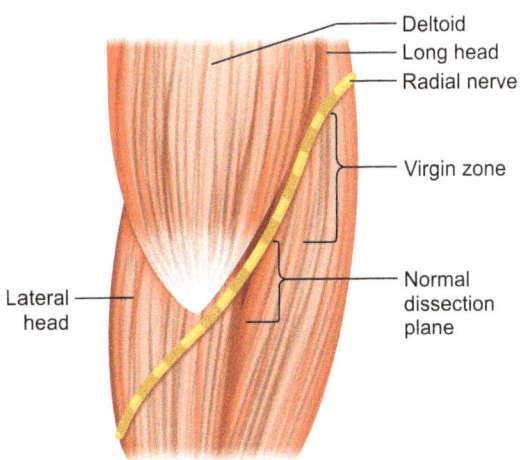

Fig. 8.14: Approach through the virgin area medially.

BROKEN NAIL REMOVAL

Broken nails can be encountered with two scenarios—(1) when the fracture has not united and (2) when the fracture has united.

Remove the proximal end first by using the appropriate nail extractor jigs and slap hammer if needed.

Most of the times the exact manufacturer and maker of an interlocking nail is not known. It is always good and safe to have a universal AO conical bolt extractor set (Fig. 8.15A) ready while attempting the nail removals. It usually takes a good hold in the threads of most of the nails. Be sure to have the thinnest size available on table.

If doing an open removal, remove distal end by holding distal end with pliers. Using nose pliers with a catch as shown in the Figure 8.15B gives a firm hold on the broken distal nail and helps removal.

When removal is attempted close, it can be done by aligning the fracture and passing special instruments under C-arm guidance. First among such instruments is a long cement

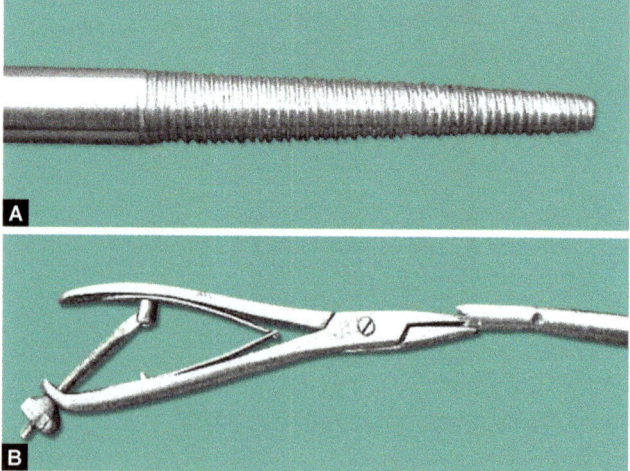

Figs. 8.15A and B: (A) Universal AO conical bolt; (B) Nose pliers with a catch.

extractor forceps of the revision total hip replacement (THR) set. On passing through the proximal medulla and fracture site, it can be used to hold and remove the broken distal end like shown in the Figure 8.16.

Another useful instrument is a hooked guidewire (Figs. 8.17A and B). After negotiating through the proximal fragment and the fracture, it can be passed through or outside the cavity of the nail. The hooked portion can be engaged at the distal end of the broken nail. The nail can be slowly back hammered with hooked guidewire using a T handle and extracted. This hooked wire has to be premade by machines and not done on OT table, as it needs acute curve which cannot be done on OT table.

Many times after removal of the proximal broken nail, the fracture is angulated. Removal of the broken end through

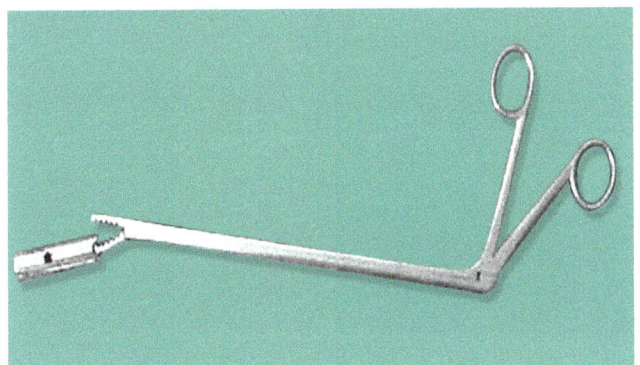

Fig. 8.16: Long cement extractor forceps of the revision total hip replacement (THR) set.

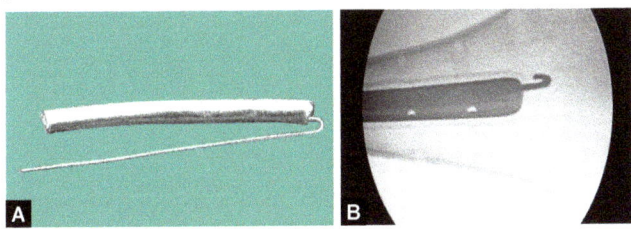

Figs. 8.17A and B: Hooked guidewire.

the angulation is difficult. A special instrument like in the Figures 8.18A and B can be used. It is passed through the proximal fragment. Using its 90° handle, the proximal and distal fragments can be aligned. The hooked guidewire can then be passed and the distal end extracted.

Another method of extracting the broken end is making an oblique hole from the outer cortex to the distal end of the nail. A beaded guidewire is passed, entering the nail with the plain end of guidewire first. Then it is maneuvered through the broken distal nail, the fracture, proximal fragment, and coming out through the entry point. The beaded tip engages at the distal end of the nail and can be used to extract out the broken nail as shown in the Figure 8.19.

If the nail has been dynamized and the distal screws have been removed, many times bone fills up the screw holes of the nail as is evident in the Figure 8.20.

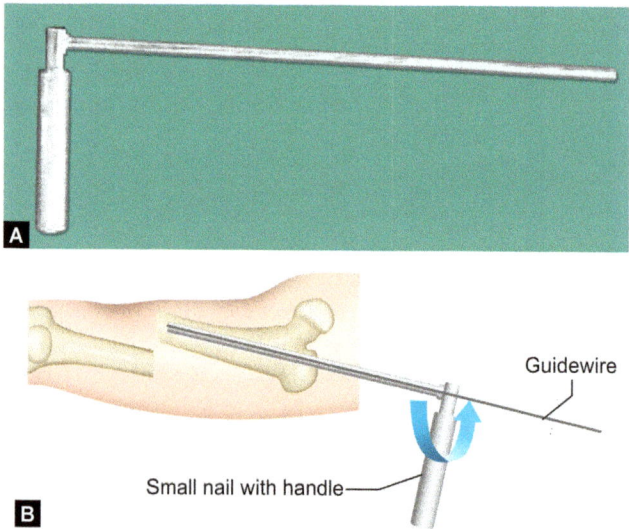

Figs. 8.18A and B: Special instrument used to align the fracture and access the broken implant in the distal fragment.

Chapter 8: Implant Removal

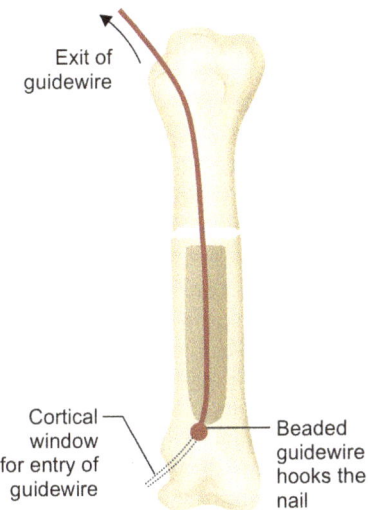

Fig. 8.19: Oblique cortical window and beaded guidewire used to extract the broken nail.

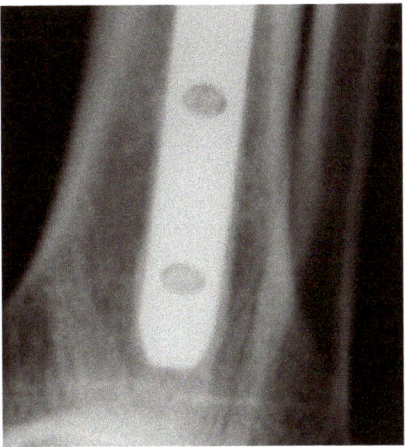

Fig. 8.20: Bony ingrowth visible in the empty distal locking bolts of the nail.

These bony ingrowths might hamper the nails from coming out. They need to be identified. The bone blocks can be broken by using thin Steinmann pins under C-arm guidance and then the nail can be easily extracted.

A few instances are encountered when a broken screw is lodged at one end of the nail, blocking it from being extracted. Its head and the proximal shaft are broken, rendering it not approachable for direct removal.

Like shown in the Figure 8.21, nail is stuck in the broken part of the screw. Method here is to drill an appropriate size Steinmann pin though the proximal hole and align it with the broken end of screw. The Steinmann is drilled with the nail sliding over Steinmann pin, and is dislodged from the broken screw and can now be extracted.

Many times, despite the best of efforts, the broken distal end of nail is difficult to get hold of and does not come out. A useful instrument in such situations is broken nail extractor reamer (Figs. 8.22A and B). It can be passed intramedullary and using the flutes on the instrument, it is rotated in an anti-clockwise

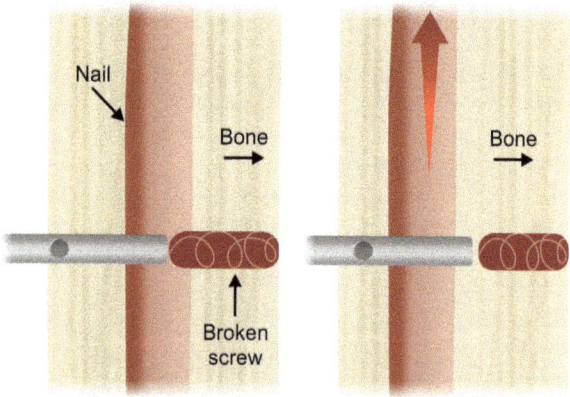

Fig. 8.21: Steinmann pin used to dislodge the nail from the broken end of the screw.

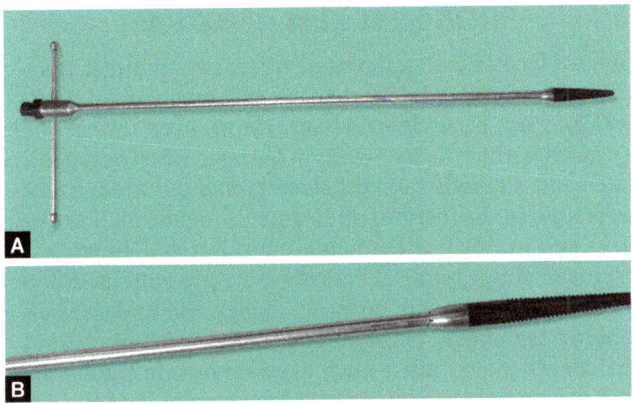

Figs. 8.22A and B: (A) Broken nail extractor reamer; (B) Reverse cutting flutes at the tip.

direction to carve out threads in the broken nail. The broken end gets subsequently held in the instrument and can be tapped or hammered out. One point to remember while using it is the tip is made of comparatively delicate material and can break if an undue mediolateral stress is applied.

BROKEN SCREW REMOVAL

Problems faced while removal of screw are multiple. The slot for the screw driver in head might become spoiled and the driver may not fit in. Special instruments, even Indian made, are available which form threads in the head when engaged and rotated anti-clockwise and the screw comes out when it takes a proper hold in the instrument (Figs. 8.23 and 8.24). If the head breaks and the shaft is left behind, it is a tricky situation. The AO broken screw removal set comes handy with its different instruments for specific purposes. When the broken shaft of the screw is outside the bone and available for some kind of hold, special pliers with a catch like as shown in Figures 8.25A and B can be used to remove it. Otherwise a hollow mill needs

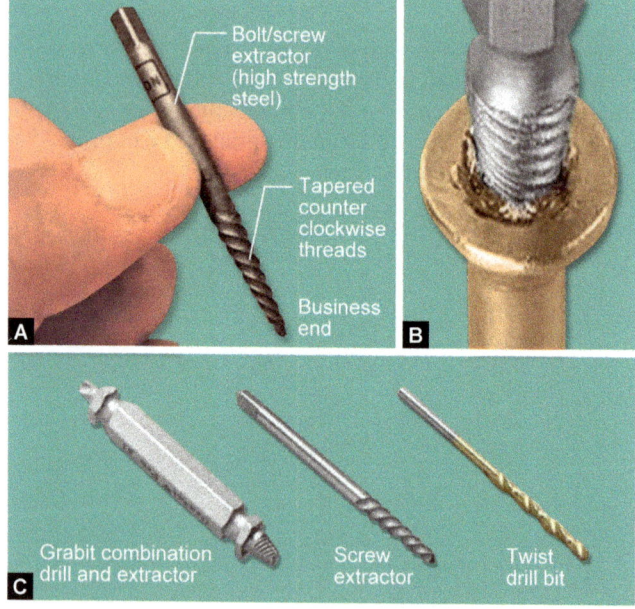

Figs. 8.23A to C: Various broken nail removal instruments.

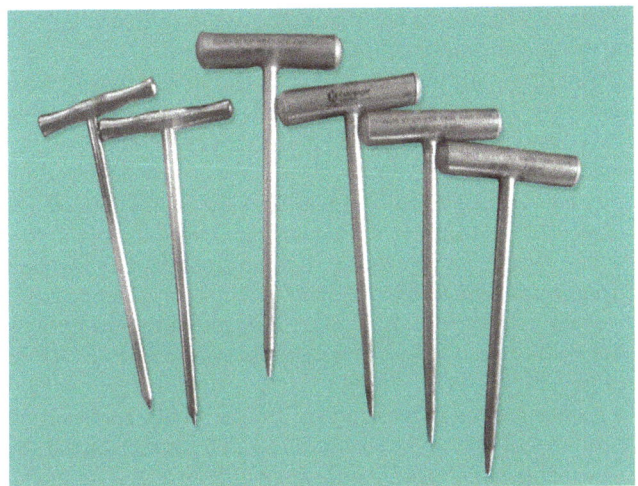

Fig. 8.24: Instruments useful when the screw head is spoiled.

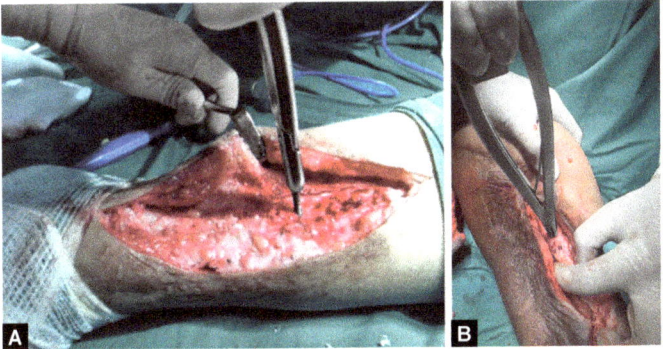

Figs. 8.25A and B: Pliers with catch to hold the shafts of a broken screw.

to be used to remove the bone around the screw and extract it by holding it with the special clamps. If the screw is deeply embedded and still cannot be removed, the opposite cortex bone around the screw might also need to be hollow milled to extract it from the opposite end.

Now let's discuss a few interesting cases to throw light on some of the tricks and methods discussed above.

- While doing an implant removal, the locking screw head gave way. The head was still locked in the plate. Two screws gave way in this manner, rest of them came out. Even the reverse cutting screw removal special instruments could not remove them. Using a high speed burr, the head was burred off (Figs. 8.26A and B), so it was dislodged from the plate. Now with all the other screws out of the plate, the plate was bent over the last screw. The plate itself was used as a lever and the screw was taken out of the bone. The remnant screw from the bone was then removed using special pliers and hollow mills (Figs. 8.27 to 8.30).

- A nonunion intertrochanteric fracture with trochanteric fixation nail system (TFN) *in situ*. The TFN broke from the area where the distal locking bolt was put (Fig. 8.31). Removing the proximal part and the neck screws was the easier part. The distal fragment was now a free fragment. First a screw was inserted into this broken piece through the static hole so that it prevents the piece from rotating or migrating distally. A guidewire was then inserted proximally. The guidewire would not go into the nail due to bone formation just where the nail

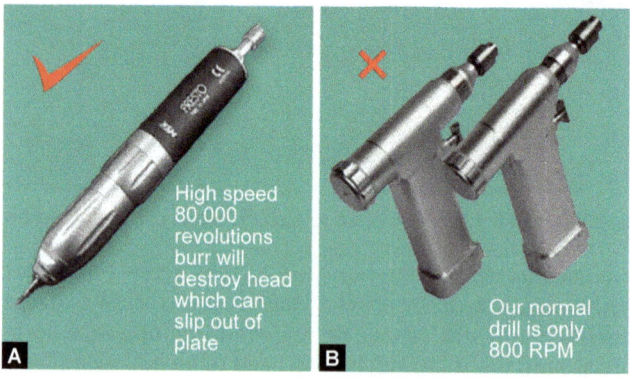

Figs. 8.26A and B: High speed burrs used to shave off the screw head.

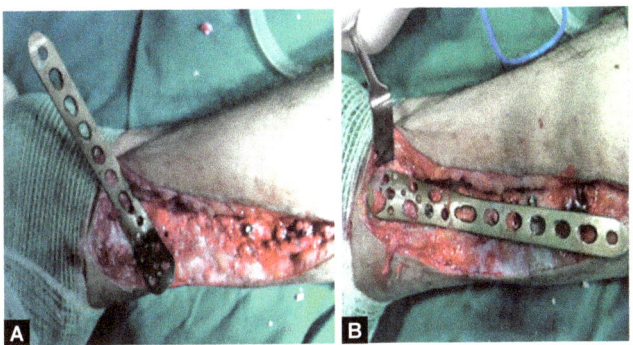

Figs. 8.27A and B: (A) Plate bent over the spoilt screw; (B) Bent plate used as a lever to rotate and take out the spoiled screw from bone.

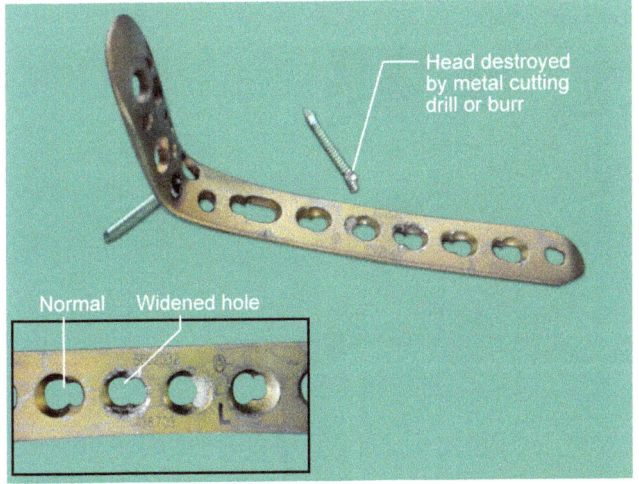

Fig. 8.28: Burred head of screw and bent plate after removal.

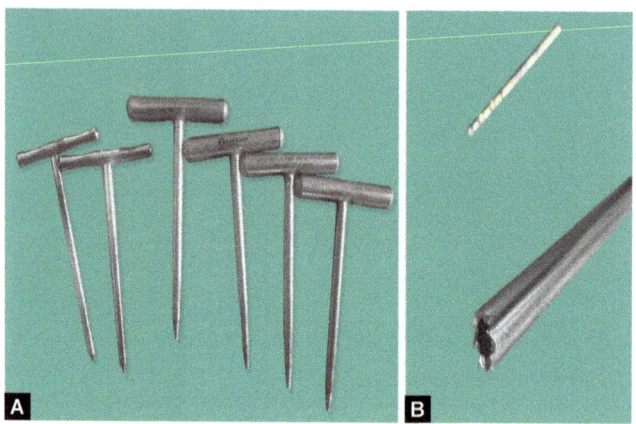

Figs. 8.29A and B: (A) Special screw removal instruments; (B) Carbide tip drill and hollow mill.

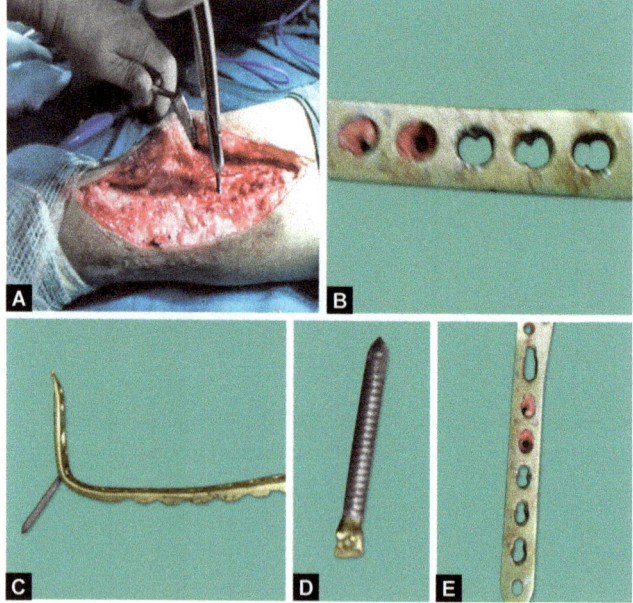

Figs. 8.30A to E: Removed broken screws and plate.

Chapter 8: Implant Removal

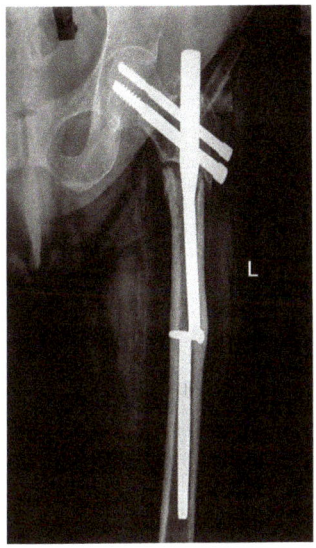

Fig. 8.31: Short proximal femoral nailing (PFN) with nail broken at shaft locking bolt.

had broken. Hence the canal was reamed to a diameter larger than the size of the nail to remove this bone. Then a broken nail implant remover instrument was used to cut flutes into it, hold it and extract it after taking out the screw which we had put into it (Figs. 8.32 to 8.37).

- Subtrochanteric fracture, primary fracture was fixed with angled blade plate. Nonunion and implant failure resulted (Figs. 8.38A to E). Second surgery was revised and fixed with 95° dynamic condylar screw (DCS) but no bone grafting was done even at this stage. Again implant failure (Figs. 8.39A and B). I inherited the case at this stage. Implant removal and long proximal femoral nailing (PFN) nailing was planned. After removal of the implant, while trying to pass the guidewire, there was bony block around the broken screws. The guidewire was passed till this level and the bony formation was removed with reamers. The same procedure was carried

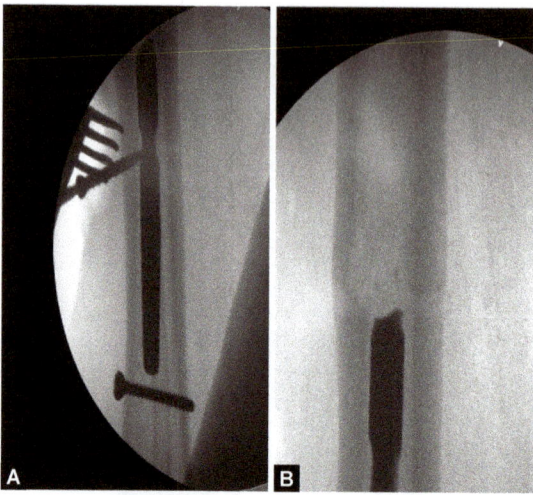

Figs. 8.32A and B: (A) Proximal part of nail was removed; (B) Problem was removal of distal broken piece.

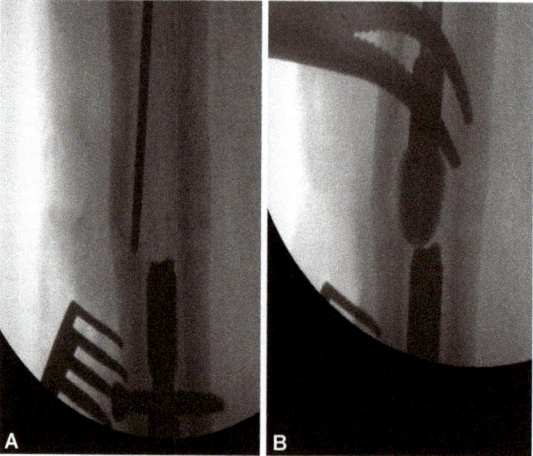

Figs. 8.33A and B: Guidewire would not go into the broken nail due to formation of bone just proximal to the broken end; (B) Hence the bone was first removed with a reamer.

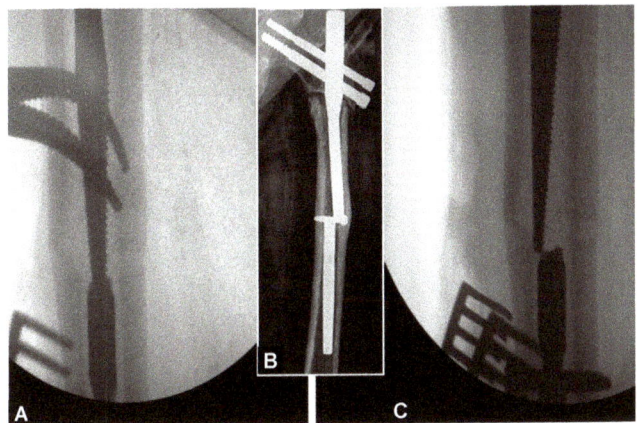

Figs. 8.34A to C: Broken nail removal instrument was used and the broken piece could be extracted.

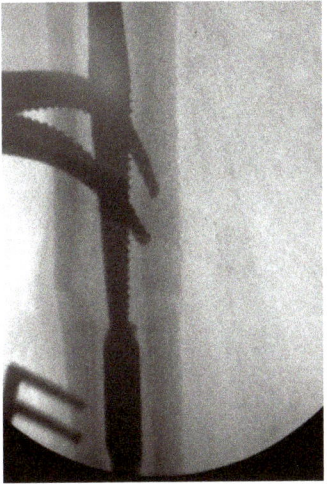

Fig. 8.35: Broken distal nail engaged in reverse flutes of special nail removal instrument.

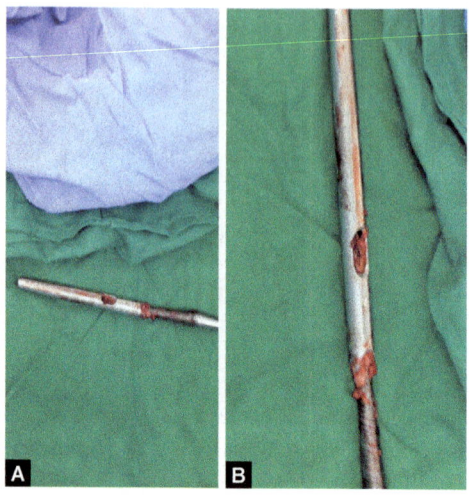

Figs. 8.36A and B: Broken nail after removal.

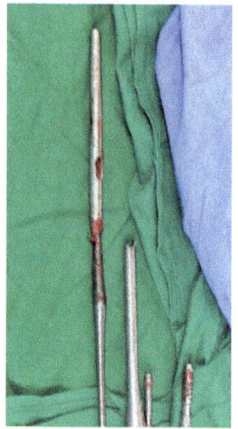

Fig. 8.37: All the removed broken implants.

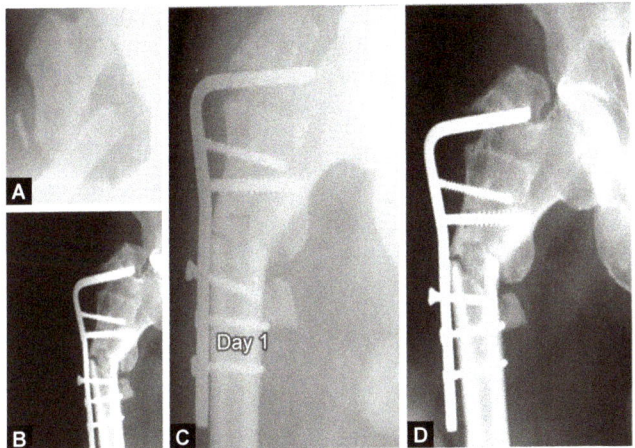

Figs. 8.38A to D: Subtrochanteric femur fracture. Fixed angle blate done initially, which went into nonunion.

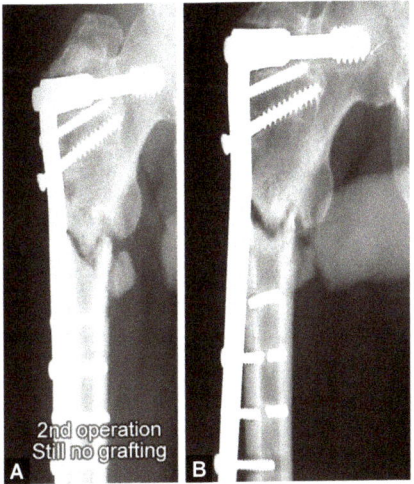

Figs. 8.39A and B: (A) Second surgery with 95° dynamic condylar screw (DCS) without bone grafting; (B) Again nonunion and implant failure.

out at each screw level and eventually the guidewire could be passed (Figs. 8.40 to 8.44). After doing a long PFN, bone grafting was done along the medial side. The fracture went on to heal subsequently.

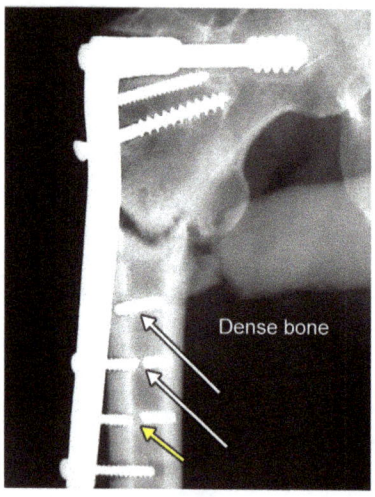

Fig. 8.40: Bone formation around periphery of the broken screws.

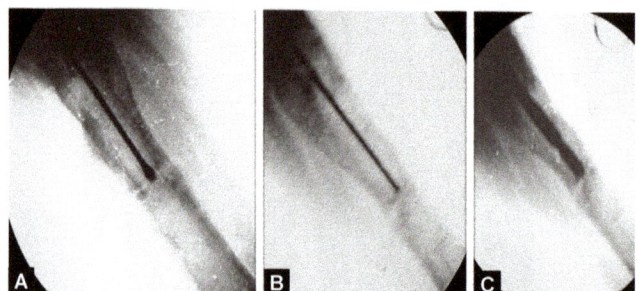

Figs. 8.41A to C: While trying to nail, guidewire could not be passed into the femur canal. Notice formation of bone along the screw tract. Guidewire was pushed till the tract and reamed with the reamer.

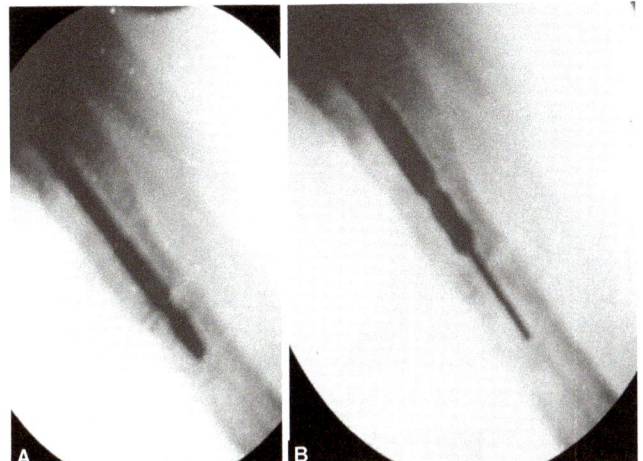

Figs. 8.42A and B: Same procedure was repeated at every subsequent screw site.

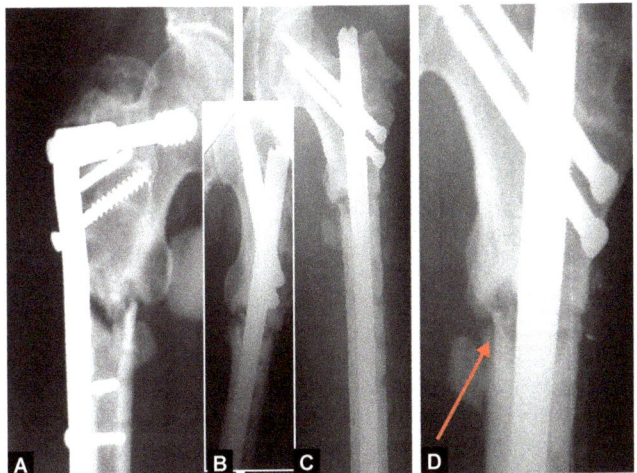

Figs. 8.43A to D: (A) Preoperative image; (B to D) Postoperative image. Long proximal femoral nailing (PFN) done with bone grafting along the medial cortex.

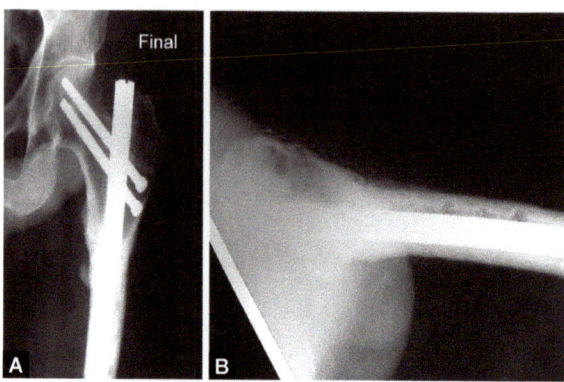

Figs. 8.44A and B: (A) A.P. and (B) Lateral views showing fracture union.

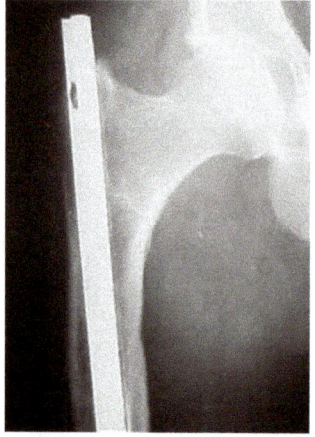

Fig. 8.45: Femur with K nail *in situ*.

- Removal of embedded K nails.
  The use of K nails for femur nailing has reduced substantially in the recent past but once in a while you do get an impacted K nail for removal. It can be removed with the hooked K nail extractors which lodge onto proximal eye of the nail and extract it (Fig. 8.45). One should be prepared with

3–4 extractors as their tips are slender and may break while trying to extract. Also the smallest size extractors should be available on table due to variation in sizes and implant design of various manufacturers. Often it happens especially if the K nail has been there for a very long duration that it is embedded in the femoral cortex distally as seen in the Figures 8.46A and B. This happens probably because it is a straight implant and not a curved one as our modern femur nails. Now to extract it we need to open a small cortical window near the distal end of the nail under C-arm guidance and free the bone around the distal end of the nail. Also we need to clear the bony ingrowth inside the distal eye of the K nail. Once this is achieved using the proximal extractors we slap hammer it out. It may not come in one go. Several cycles of hammering it in and out might help us eventually achieve the removal.

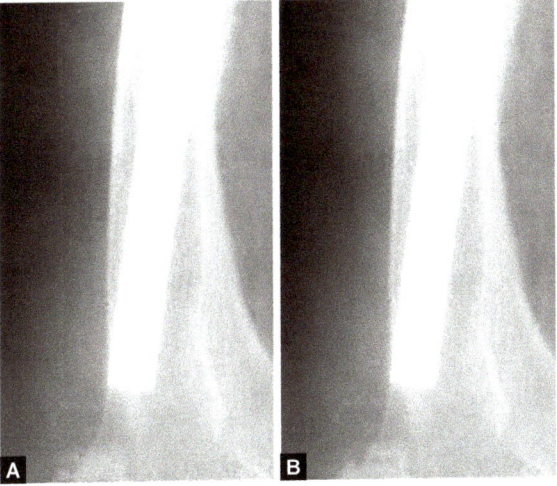

Figs. 8.46A and B: Distal end of the nail is embedded in the cortex.

Chapter 9

Interesting Cases

DD Tanna

CASE 1: UNDISPLACED FEMUR NECK FRACTURE

A 71-year-old female was presented with complaint of pain in left hip since 10 days when walking full weight bearing. X-ray report showed no fracture but I was not completely convinced. In suspected femur neck fractures, you should always order internal rotation views. Portable X-ray in ward with limb lying in external rotation is not a decision-making X-ray report. Internal rotation view shows the fracture as shown in Figures 9.1A and B.

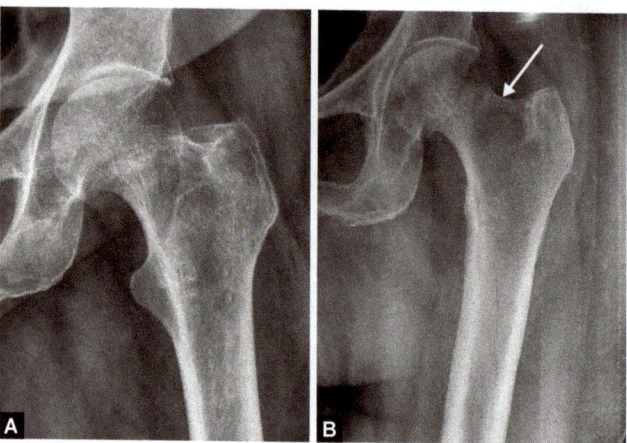

Figs. 9.1A and B: (A) X-ray says no #. Not convinced with the X-ray; (B) You must order internal rotation view. Portable poor X-ray image when limb lying in external rotation is not a definitive decision making X-ray. Internal rotation view X-ray shows fracture in B.

Another example: An old-age female presenting with pain in left hip. X-ray report is normal. Clinically, it is a fractured hip. For all practical purposes, there is nothing like sprain of hip. Internal rotation view was taken, still no fracture was seen (Fig. 9.2). Based on my strong clinical suspicion for an unexplained pain, I ordered MRI scan. MRI report suggested fracture (Figs. 9.3A and B). Going back to X-ray A, now in hind site we can suspect

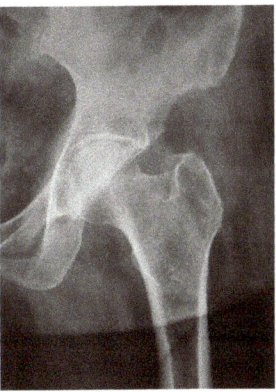

Fig. 9.2: History of fall. Pain in hip, clinically its fracture hip. There is nothing like sprain of hip for all practical aspects. X-ray normal. How do you explain the pain.

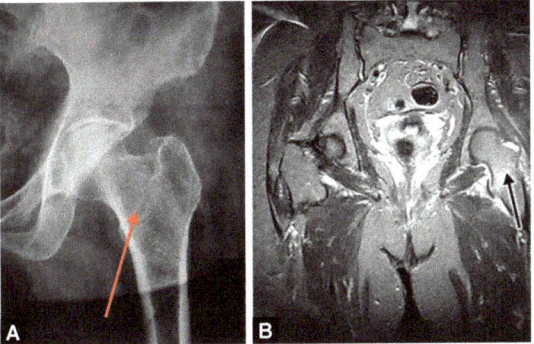

Figs. 9.3A and B: (A) X-ray which is reported normal; (B) MRI report suggests fracture. Going back to X-ray (A), now in hind sight we can suspect fracture.

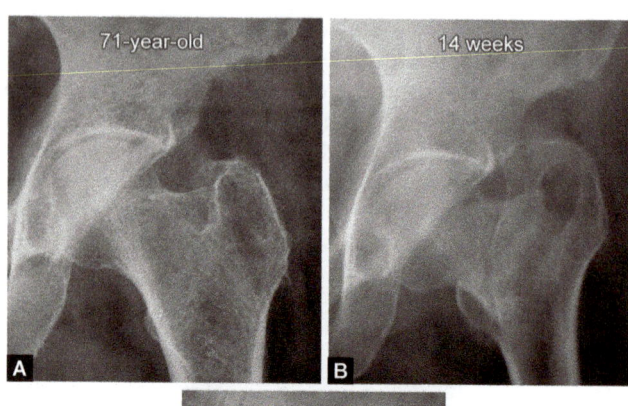
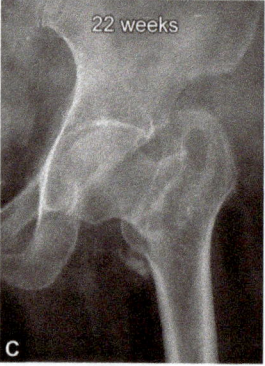

Figs. 9.4A to C: 71-year-old patient did not get convinced with MRI proof of fracture. She did not see fracture in X-ray. She refused surgery; (A) At presentation; (B) At 14 weeks; and (C) At 22 weeks X-rays shows deterioration of the fracture.

fracture. I was convinced about the fracture and advised surgery to the patient. Patient was not convinced with MRI proof; she did not see fracture in X-ray report. Hence, she refused surgery. X-ray reports in subsequent months showed deterioration of the fracture. If it was treated early, it could have been fixed (Figs. 9.4A to C). Ultimately, she had to undergo hip hemi replacement (Figs. 9.5A to D). So take home message here is:

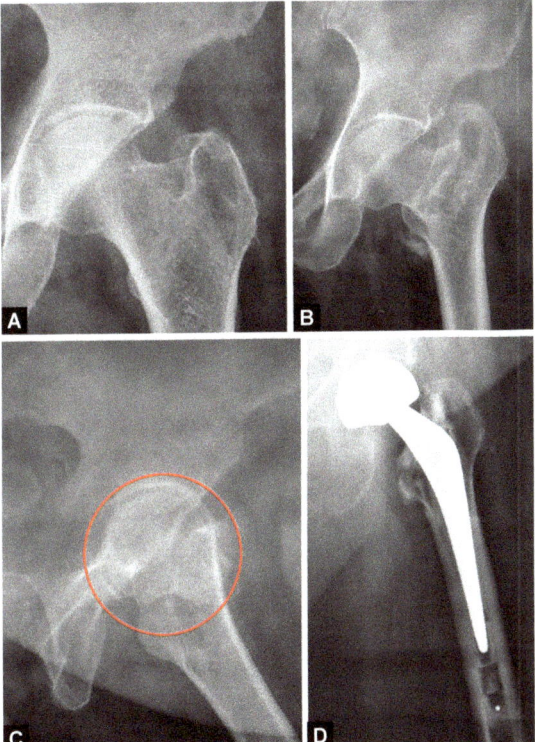

Figs. 9.5A to D: If treated early it could have been fixed. Ultimately, she had to undergo hip replacement surgery; (A) Original injury; (B and C) 6 months later; (D) After replacement.

- X-ray of suspected neck femur if normal, is *not* definite.
- X-ray report of the wet portable film by radiologist is very dicey.
- Internal rotation view is must. If no fracture is detected still and there is strong suspicion of fracture, get an MRI done.
- If MRI also shows no fracture in suspected case, it is almost final there is no fracture.

CASE 2: CONSERVATIVE TREATMENT OF FEMUR NECK FRACTURE

Transcervical fracture can be conserved in valgus impacted fracture and not in B undisplaced fracture (Figs. 9.6 and 9.7). Undisplaced fracture can be seen when the initial X-ray image is taken, it can get displaced any time (Figs. 9.8 and 9.9). Most of the femur neck fractures I prefer to go with dynamic hip screw (DHS)

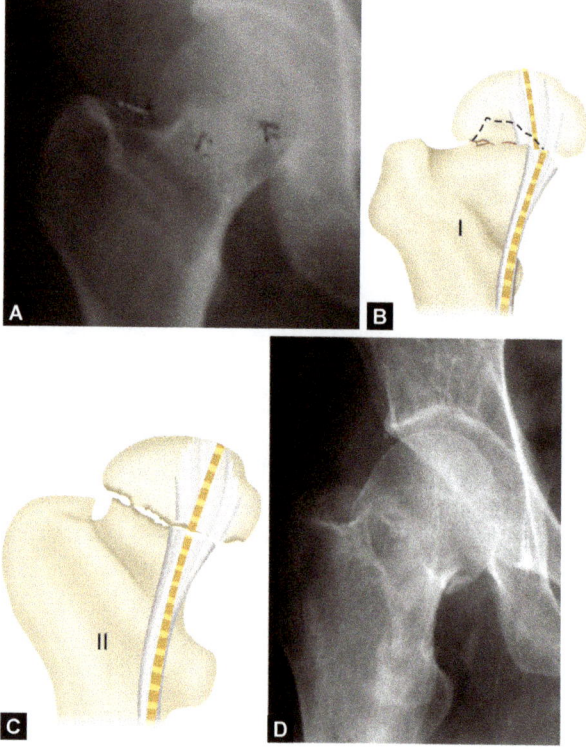

Figs. 9.6A to D: (A and B) When it can be conserved: impacted valgus fracture. Transcervical fracture can be conserved in valgus impacted fracture, and not in (C and D) undisplaced fracture. Undisplaced fracture can get displaced any time.

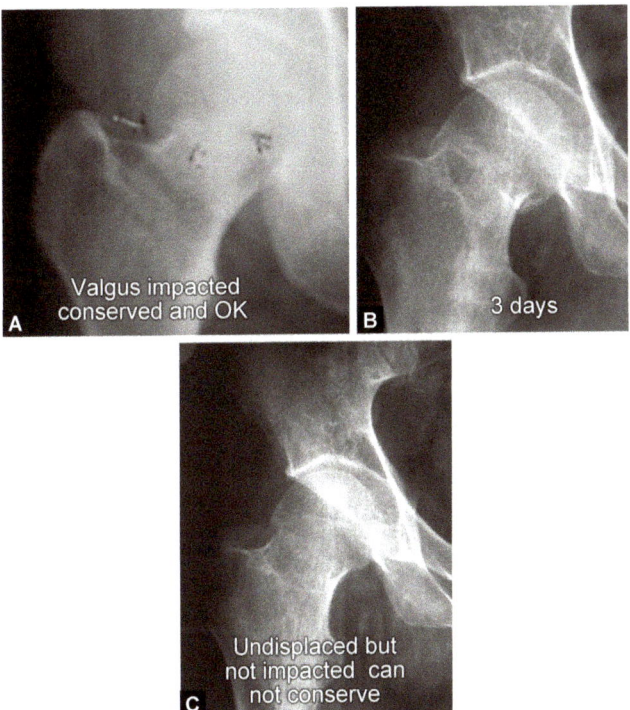

Figs. 9.7A to C: (A) Valgus impacted, most likely this will not get displaced; (B and C) This can get displaced.

and derotation screw rather than 3 C.C screws. When to conserve my rule of thumb: Valgus impacted fracture. When patient comes walking full weight bearing with little pain with patient giving history of the injury being few days old. X-ray report shows a fracture surprisingly. Now it is safe to pronounce conservative management. Same fractures, on day 1—must be fixed, and should not take a chance (Figs. 9.10A to D).

Decision is not whether to conserve or not, decision is which surgery should be performed. In young patients, fix it urgently.

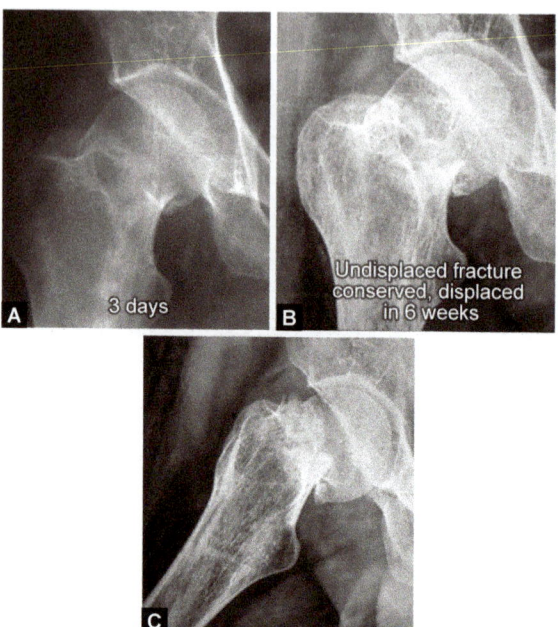

Figs. 9.8A to C: Undisplaced fracture conserved, displaced in 6 weeks. (A) X-ray at 3 days; (B and C) At 6 weeks showing displacement.

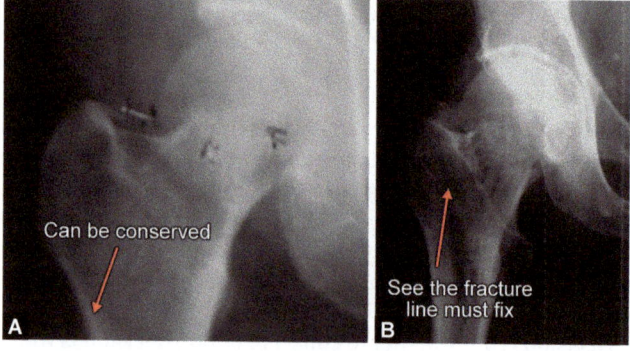

Figs. 9.9A and B: Both are valgus. (A) Is impacted in valgus and stable; (B) Is positioned in valgus but not stable.

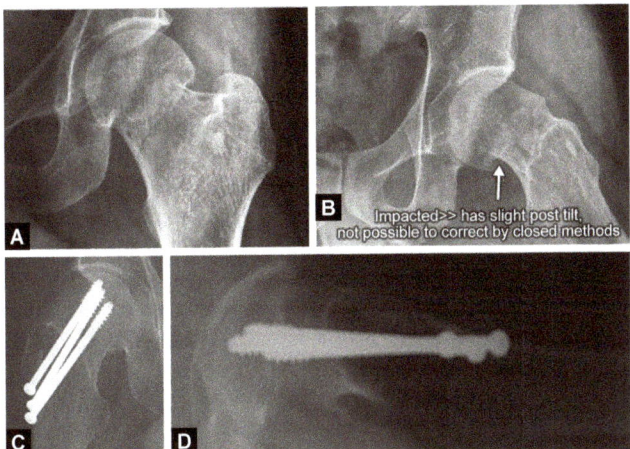

Figs. 9.10A to D: Only the valgus impacted and minimally displaced fractures with early presentation, I fix with three screws. Most others I fix with dynamic hip screw (DHS) short plate and derotation screw. (A and B) Preoperative and (C and D) Postoperative X-rays.

Delay of 24 hours or more to achieve medical stabilization have been shown not to increase morbidity or mortality. Sexson and Lehner also found that early surgery was detrimental to medically unstable, elderly patients with hip-fracture. Many studies have shown 24 hours of delay, does not make a difference.

CASE 3: WADDLING GAIT

Patient was presented with waddling gait and difficulty in walking for few weeks. X-ray report of pelvis was normal (Fig. 9.11). My conclusion was that one cannot have waddling gait without any problem. A digital X-ray image of both the hips with upper half femur was done. Stress fracture was seen (Fig. 9.12) on both sides. Calcium, vitamin D and rest will heal fractures. Insufficiency fracture, in our language stress fracture needs vitamin D3 level estimation, bone densitometry (DEXA) scan. Or be practical and give 1,500 mg daily calcium + vitamin D3 without investigations and see Figure 9.13, stress fractures heals up without any surgery.

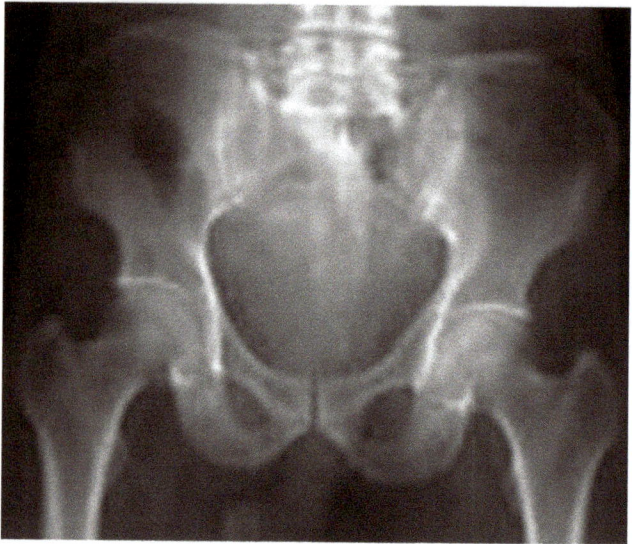

Fig. 9.11: Waddling gait and difficulty in walking. X-ray pelvis is normal. Cannot have waddling gait without any problem.

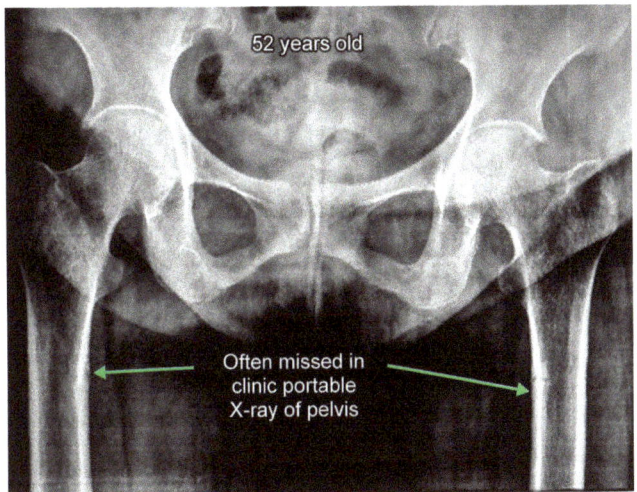

Fig. 9.12: Stress fracture seen on both sides. Calcium, vitamin D and rest will heal fracture and will be ok.

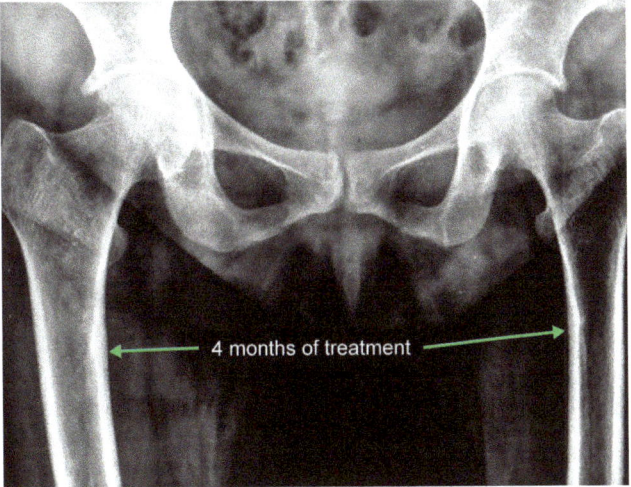

Fig. 9.13: After 4 months of treatment.

IDIOPATHIC OSTEOPOROSIS OF HEAD OF FEMUR (FIGS. 9.14A AND B)

This is not avascular necrosis (AVN). There is no epiphyseal lesion that shows such diffuse signal changes. It needs no

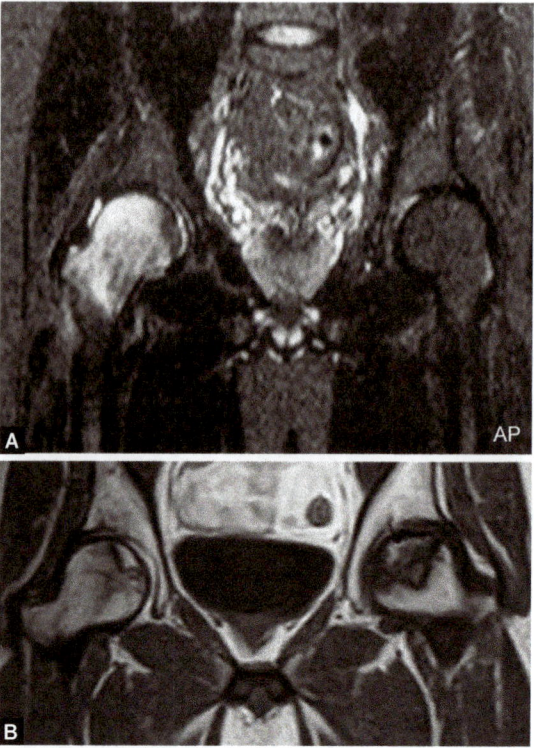

Figs. 9.14A and B: (A) This is not avascular necrosis (AVN). There is no isolated epiphyseal lesion. This is a very diffuse signal change. Needs no treatment except calcium and vitamin D3; (B) Localized epiphyseal lesion like this needs core decompression at earliest for aborting more involvement of head. For whatever it is worth.

treatment except for calcium and vitamin D3. Now it is understood as insufficiency fractures. This is also called idiopathic osteoporosis of head of femur (Figs. 9.15A and B).

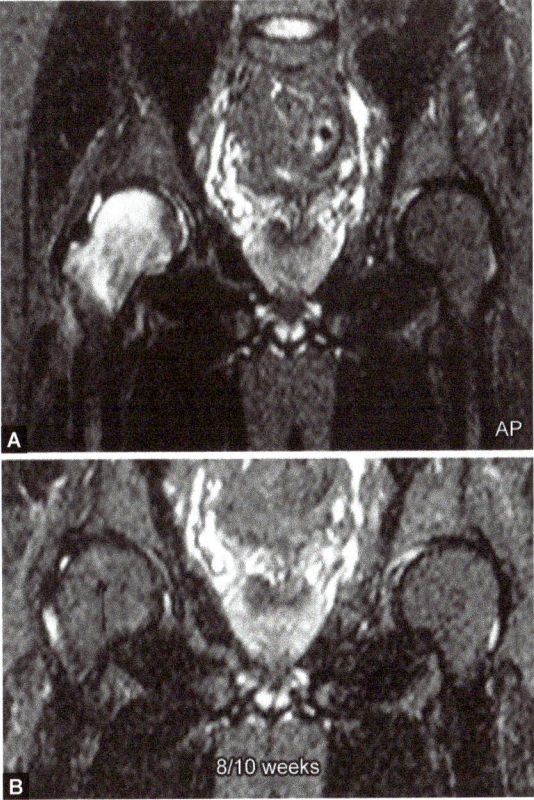

Figs. 9.15A and B: Now it is understood as insufficiency fractures. This is called idiopathic osteoporosis of head of femur. (A) MRI image at presentation; (B) At 10 weeks of taking treatment, all changes reversed and patient was normal without any collapse.

TIP OF ULNA FRACTURE

This fracture is very tricky and most surgeons leave it alone as it is a small tip fracture. Actually that tip contains important central part of triceps and patient has weakness of power in elbow extension (Figs. 9.16 and 9.17).

On exploration, one can observe, on tip of the ulna piece is attached central part of triceps, which is sutured and triceps continuity is established (Figs. 9.18 to 9.21).

Figures 9.22 to 9.31 is a complete case courtesy Dr Sangeet Gawhale, which explains this very well.

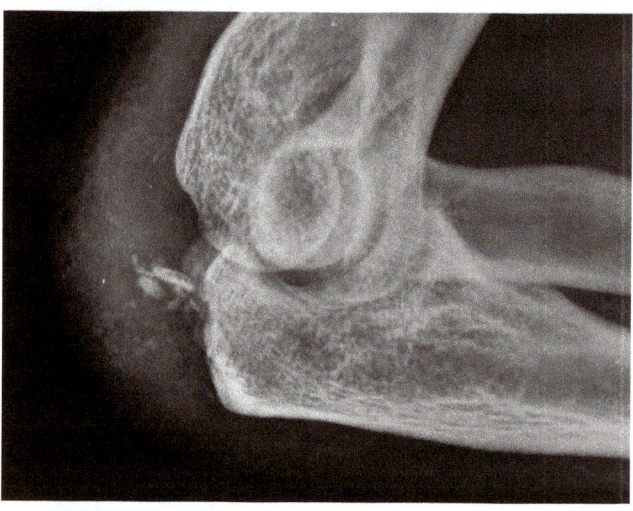

Fig. 9.16: X-ray elbow shows suspected calcified mass on tip of olecranon.

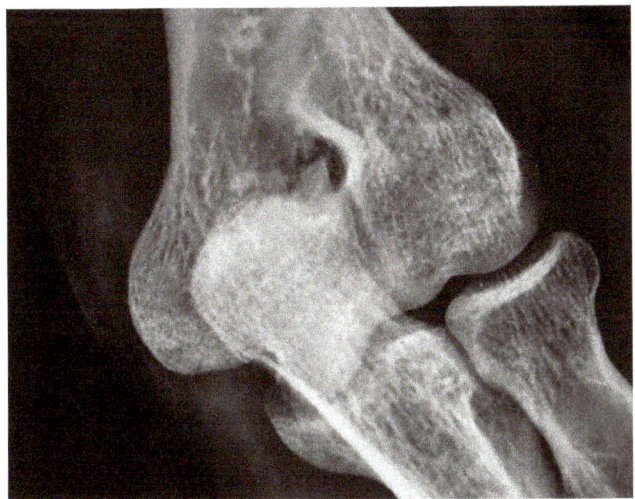

Fig. 9.17: Elbow A.P. X-ray appears near normal.

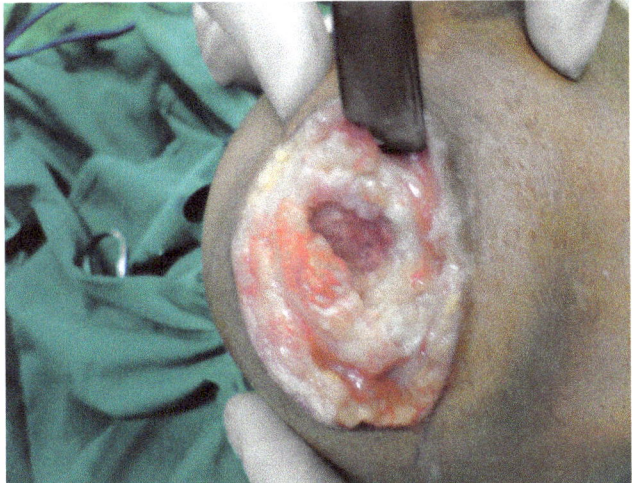

Fig. 9.18: Defect at the tip of olecranon post the avulsion.

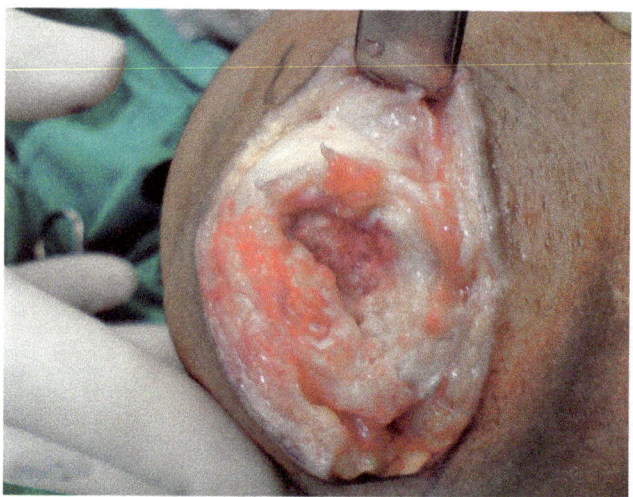

Fig. 9.19: Bony tip identified and avulsion bed cleaned, prepared for re-attachment.

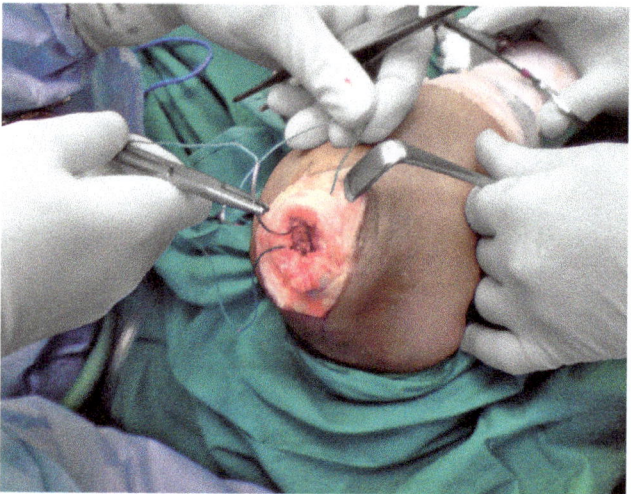

Fig. 9.20: Repair and augmented with ethibond sutures.

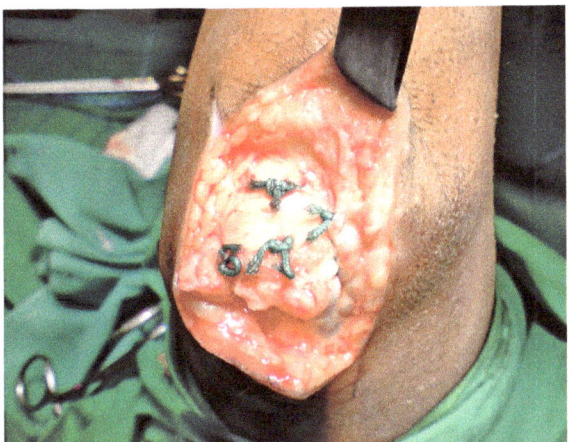

Fig. 9.21: Intraoperative picture post repair.

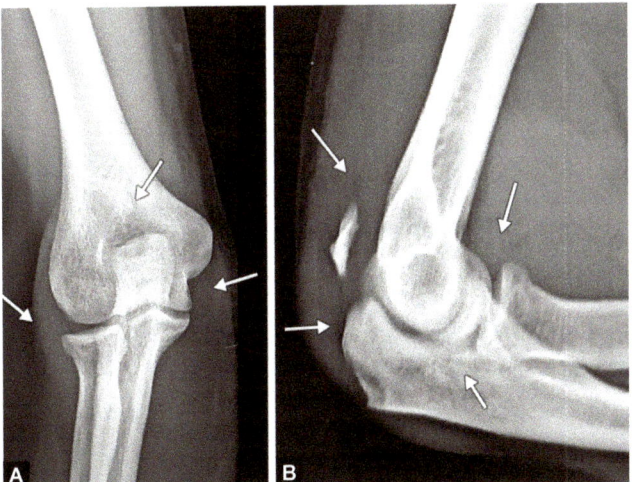

Figs. 9.22A and B: This is Dr Sangeet Gawhale's patient. 30 years old, presented with pain in elbow following a fall while playing cricket. Range of motion almost full but significant weak extension. X-ray report shows small flake of bone at olecranon tip. (A) Anteroposterior and; (B) Lateral views of elbow.

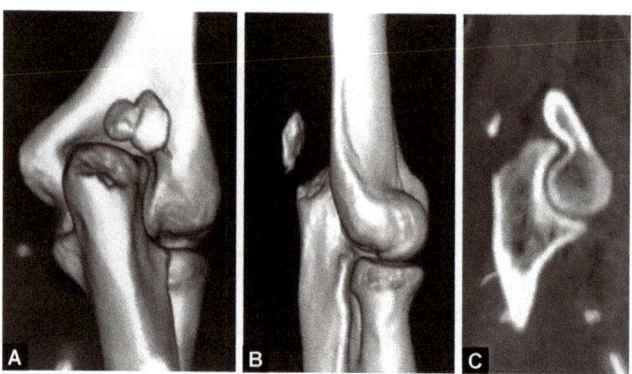

Figs. 9.23A to C: CT scan reveals large avulsed fragment from the tip of olecranon.

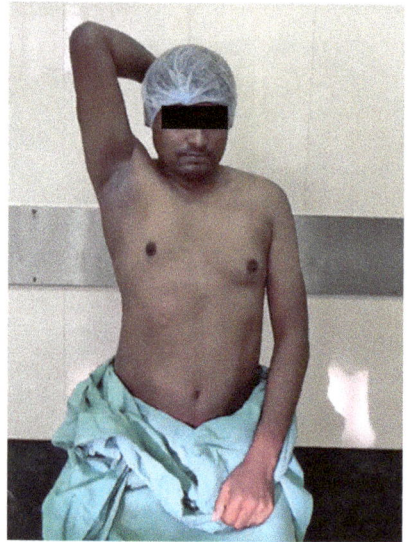

Fig. 9.24: Active extension is weak.

Chapter 9: Interesting Cases

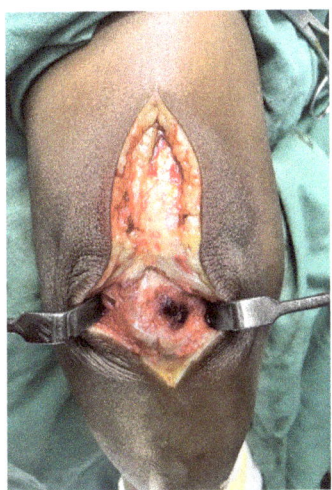

Fig. 9.25: Posterior midline incision. Defect in the tip of olecranon.

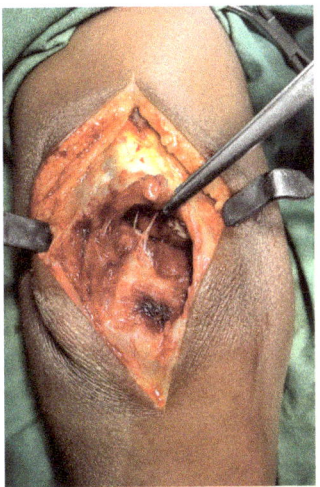

Fig. 9.26: After lifting the fragment attached to triceps significant rent along both sides of triceps is observed. The triceps is avulsed from olecranon tip along with large chunk of bone.

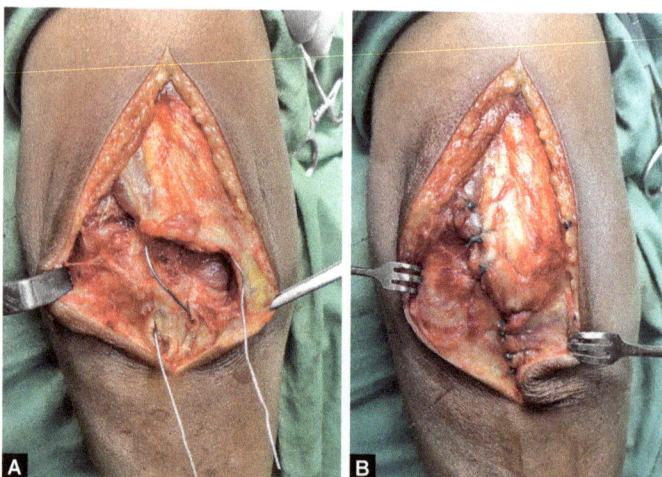

Figs. 9.27A and B: Fixation of bone fragment with Figure of 8 cerclage wire and triceps aponeurosis repair with ethibond sutures. (A) Immediately before and (B) After the complete repair.

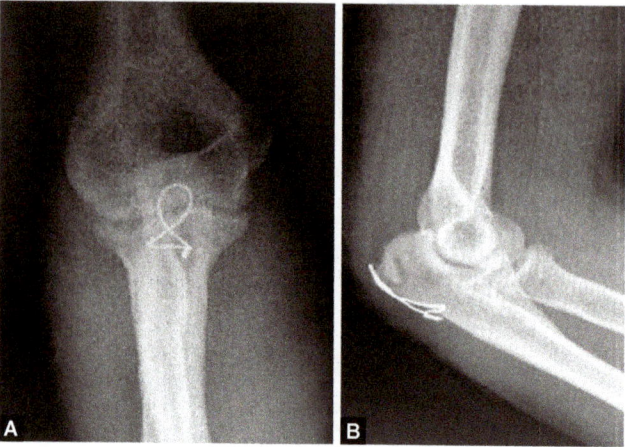

Figs. 9.28A and B: Postoperative X-ray films.

Chapter 9: Interesting Cases

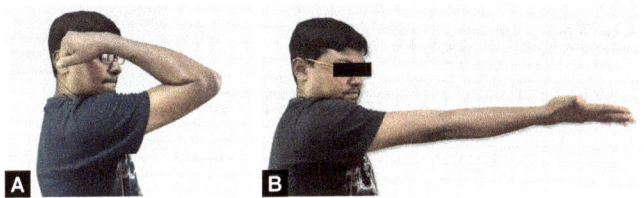

Figs. 9.29A and B: Postoperative 6 weeks: Full range of movements.

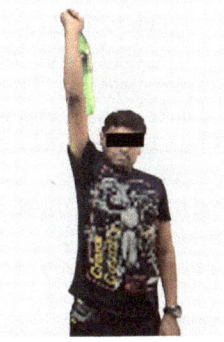

Fig. 9.30: Can lift weight easily after surgery which he could not do before surgery.

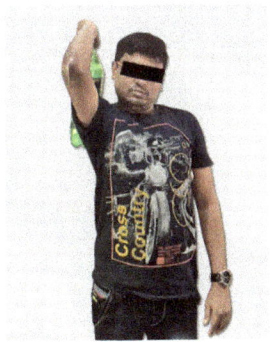

Fig. 9.31

Intramedullary Fibula for Treatment of Nonunion Long Bones

Chapter 10

DD Tanna

For management of nonunion of long bones like humerus, femur and tibia, use of an intramedullary fibula graft can be very useful. This is especially true for the atrophic variety of nonunions many times after having multiple surgeries. The fibula is harvested from the middle third of its length. Sometimes in the humerus, the fibula must be split into half to reduce its diameter due the narrow medullary space available (Figs. 10.1A and B). This can be achieved by harvesting only half of the desired length from the native site and leaving the other half intact with the parent bone (Figs. 10.2A to C). The medullary cavity at the nonunion site is

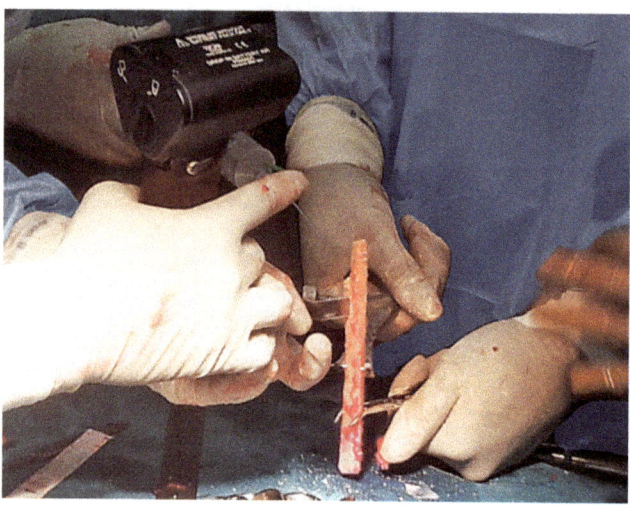

Fig. 10.1A: Harvested fibula graft.

Chapter 10: Intramedullary Fibula for Treatment of Nonunion…

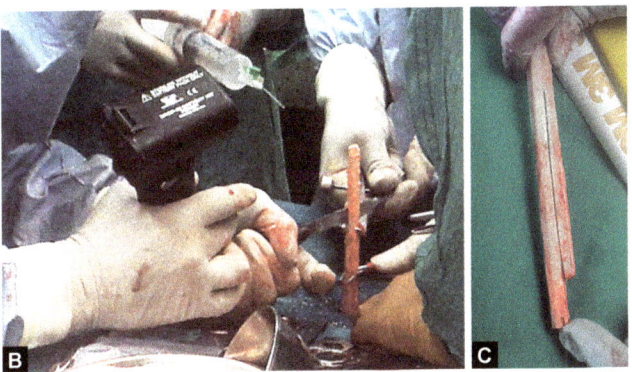

Figs. 10.1B and C: Fibula being trimmed with saw.

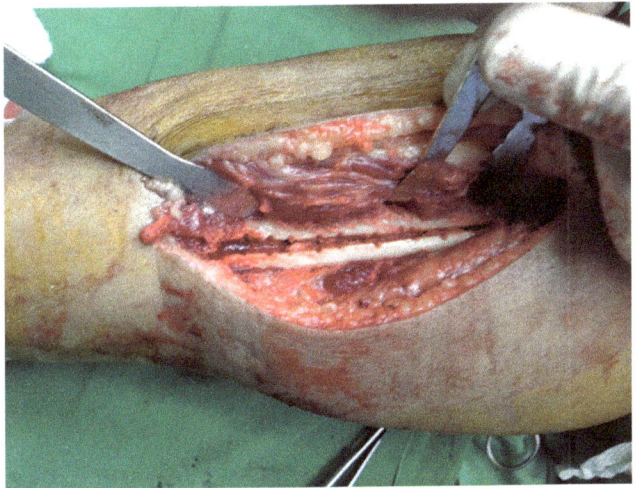

Fig. 10.2A: Intraoperative picture of half fibula graft being taken.

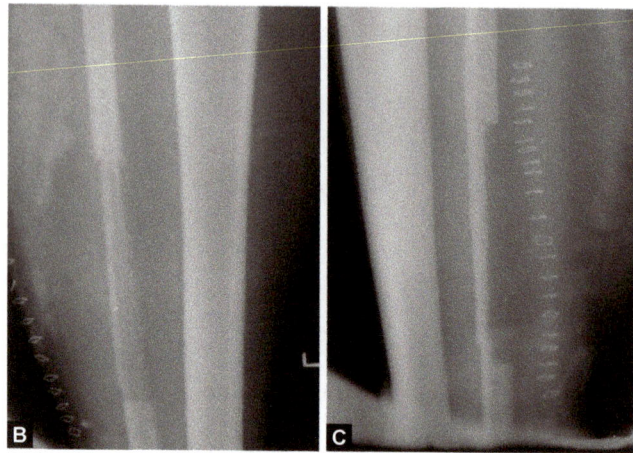

Figs. 10.2B and C: Postoperative X-ray after half fibula graft harvesting.

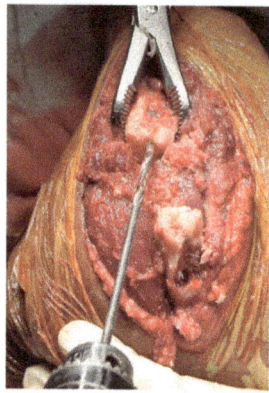

Fig. 10.3: Open up medullary cavity. Ream with gradually increasing power reamer to adequate size to fit in fibula.

opened (Fig. 10.3) and the fibula graft is inserted into it (Figs. 10.4A and B). It is preferable that the fibula moves free in the medullary cavity after insertion (Fig. 10.5). Ideally the size of the fibula graft

Chapter 10: Intramedullary Fibula for Treatment of Nonunion...

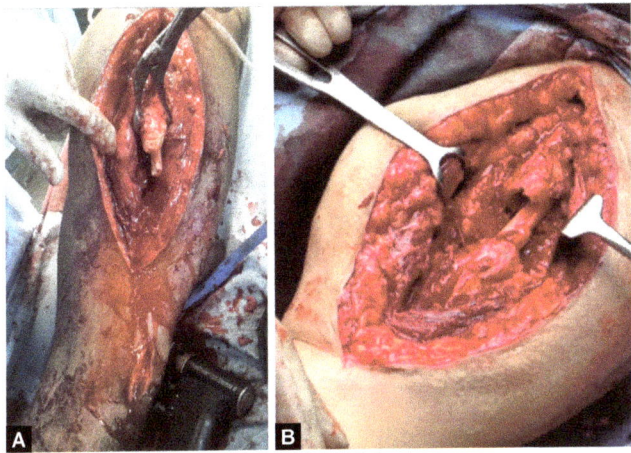

Figs. 10.4A and B: Fibula graft inserted intramedullary at nonunion site.

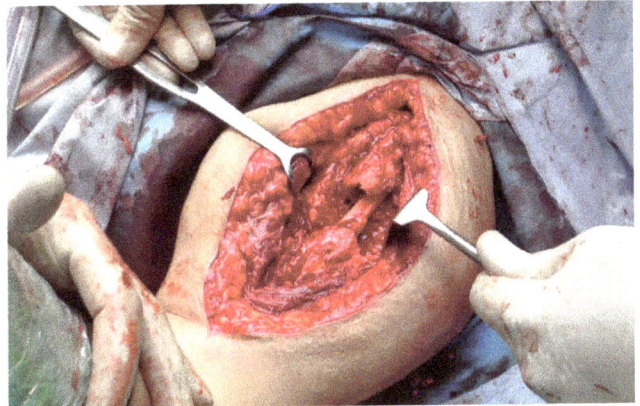

Fig. 10.5: The fibula should move freely inside the medullary cavity.

should be one smaller than the last reamer used to dilate the humeral medullary cavity. The size of fibula can be measured using the femur K nail size gauge or anterior cruciate ligament

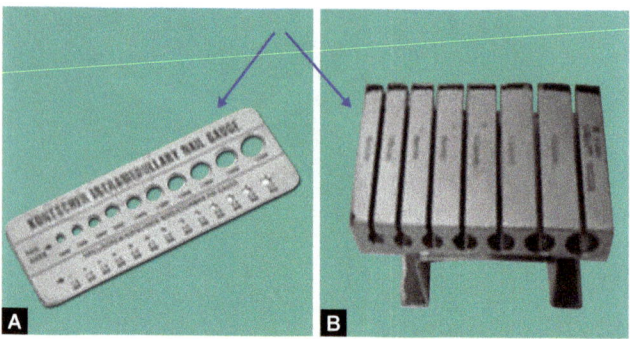

Figs. 10.6A and B: Now use. (A) K nail femur gauge or (B) Anterior cruciate ligament (ACL) graft measure sleeves to judge trimming down the fibula.

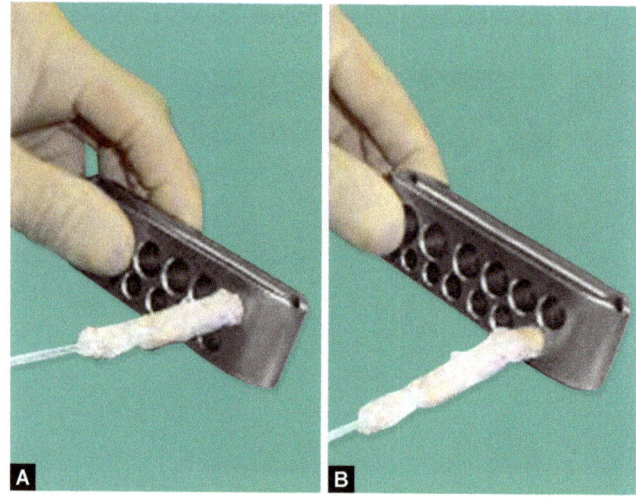

Figs. 10.7A and B: Measure the fibula.

(ACL) graft measure sleeves (Figs. 10.6 and 10.7). The graft is placed intramedullary so as to ideally have identical lengths in both the fragments. The fracture is now fixed with compression plating and massive cancellous graft (Figs. 10.8 to 10.10).

Chapter 10: Intramedullary Fibula for Treatment of Nonunion...

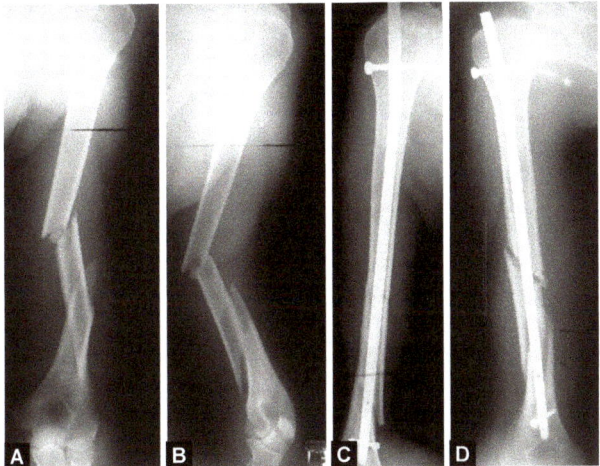

Figs. 10.8A to D: Segmental fracture humerus, treated with intramedullary nail. (A and B) Preoperative; (C and D) Postoperative X-rays.

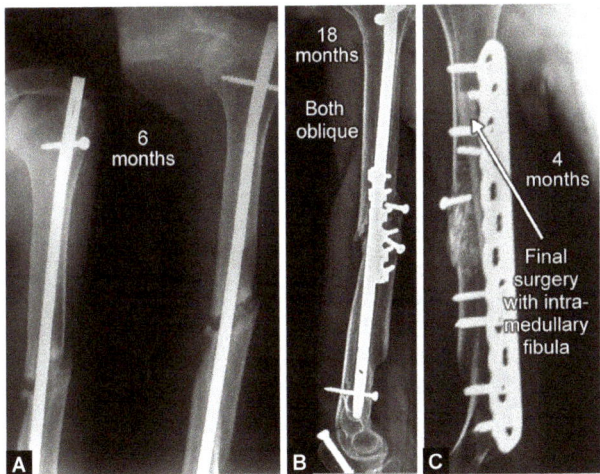

Figs. 10.9A to C: Nonunion fracture humerus treated with intramedullary fibula graft and plating. (A) At 6 months nonunion with nail inside. (B) At 18 months with nail and added plate, still nonunion. (C) Plate with intramedullary fibula healed at 4 months after third surgery.

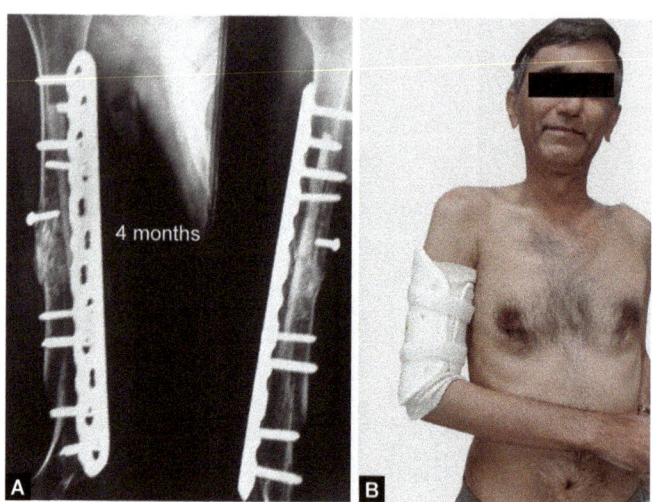

Figs. 10.10A and B: (A) Follow-up X-ray images showing union at 4 months; (B) Arm kept in a protective brace.

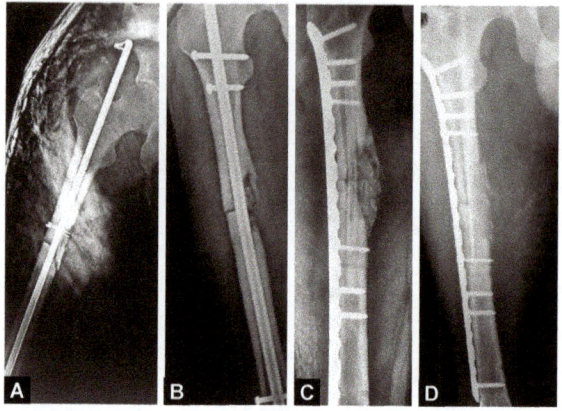

Figs. 10.11A to D: (A and B) Nonunion femur; (C and D) Treated with intramedullary fibula graft and long femur plate.

Chapter 10: Intramedullary Fibula for Treatment of Nonunion...

Fibula was used earlier for screw hold in porotic bone before the days of locking plate. Now it has the same purpose along with ostogenetic property. Few cases Figures 10.11 to 10.41 and 10.42 to 10.48.

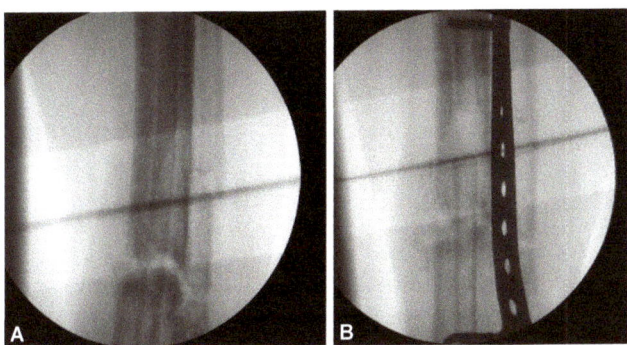

Figs. 10.12A and B: C-arm images of nonunion with. (A) Intramedullary fibula; (B) Intramedullary fibula with plate.

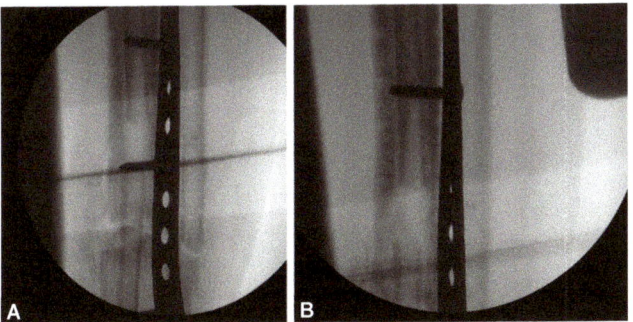

Figs. 10.13A and B: Screws passed through the fibula graft for additional stability.

144 *Orthopedic Secrets*

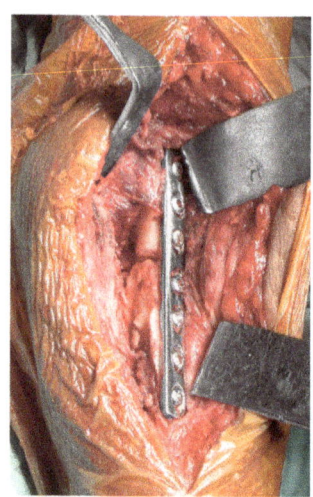

Fig. 10.14: Intraoperative image of nonunion treated with fibula graft, plating and cancellous graft.

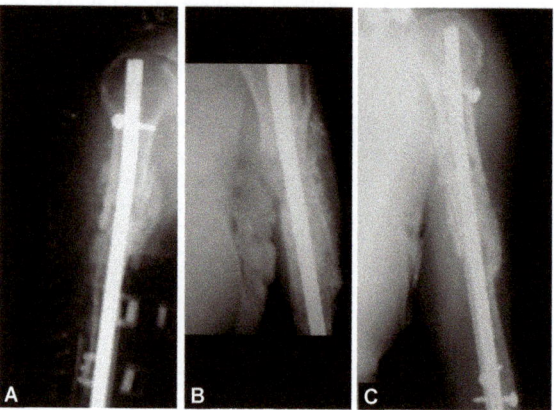

Figs. 10.15A to C: (A) Immediate postoperative; (B and C) 4 months. Things ok.

Chapter 10: Intramedullary Fibula for Treatment of Nonunion...

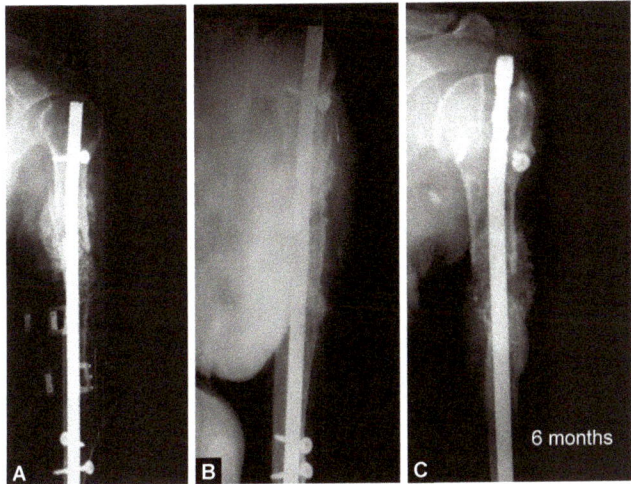

Figs. 10.16A to C: Locking nail with massive graft before days of locking plate.

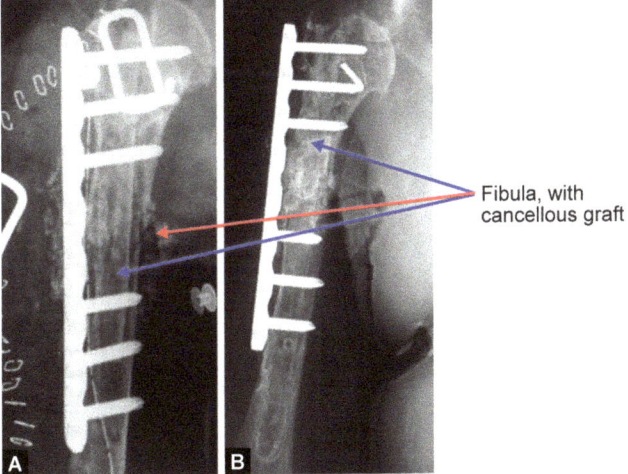

Fibula, with cancellous graft

Figs. 10.17A and B: (A) Nice locking plate with massive grafting (auto +allo) immediate postoperative; (B) 6 month united.

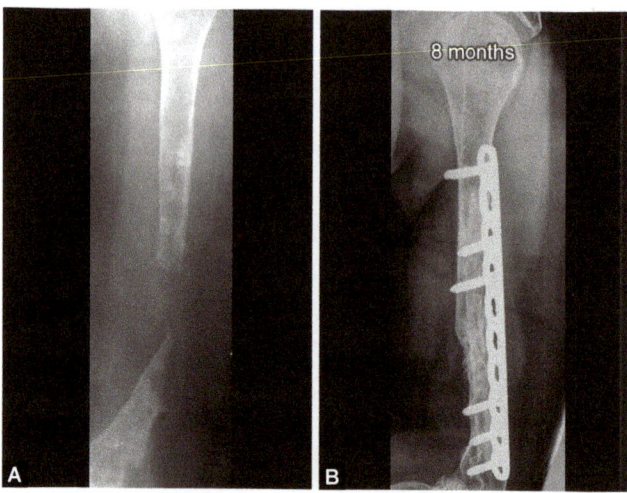

Figs. 10.18A and B: (A) Infected implant removed. 2 years no infection. 70-year-old severe porotic; (B) Had put in intramedullary fibula and shortened humerus getting compaction and locking plate.

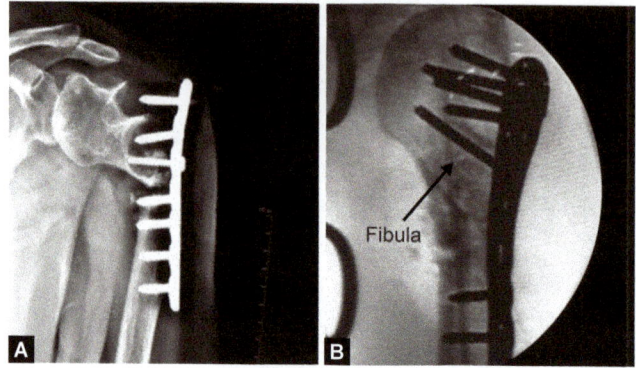

Figs. 10.19A and B: (A) Fracture surgical neck humerus, treated initially with normal dynamic compression plate (DCP), went into nonunion; (B) Intramedullary cortical strut and medial cancellous grafting with philos plating done.

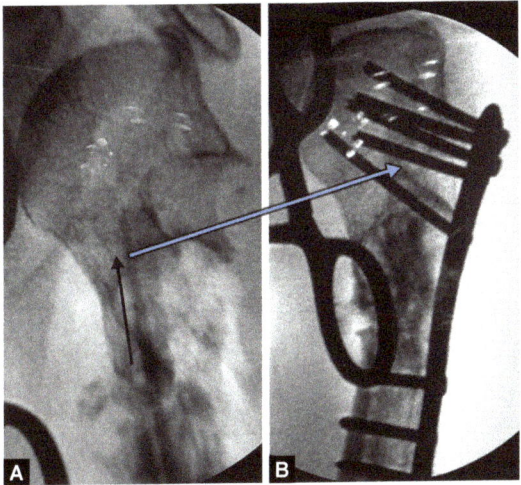

Figs. 10.20A and B: (A) Intramedullary fibula with massive cancellous bone graft; (B) With added philos plate.

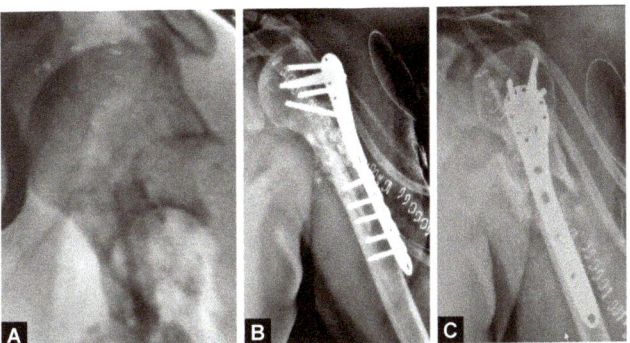

Figs. 10.21A to C: Immediate postoperative X-ray images.

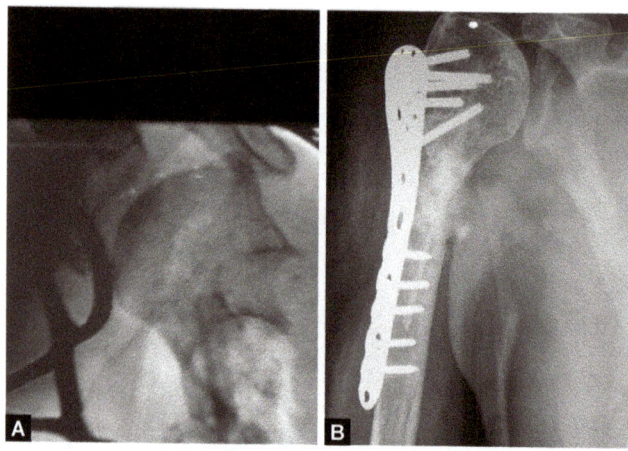

Figs. 10.22A and B: Another similar example. (A) Intraoperative; (B) Postoperative showing union at fracture site.

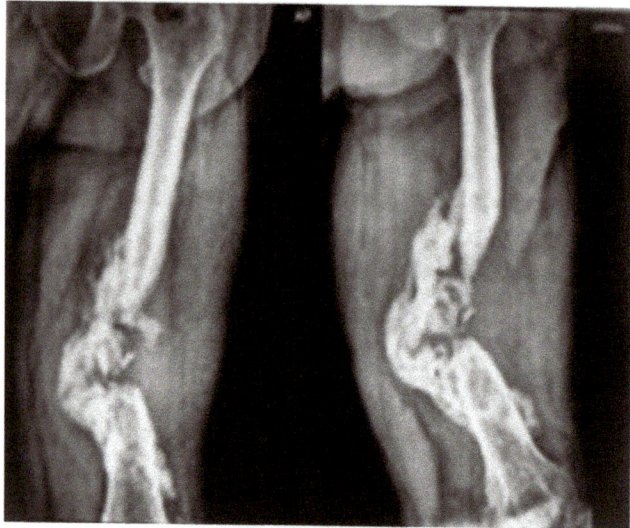

Fig. 10.23: 48 years old patient. 3 years after index surgery, undergone five surgeries. Sequestrectomy infection control, no sinus since 1 year.

Chapter 10: Intramedullary Fibula for Treatment of Nonunion...

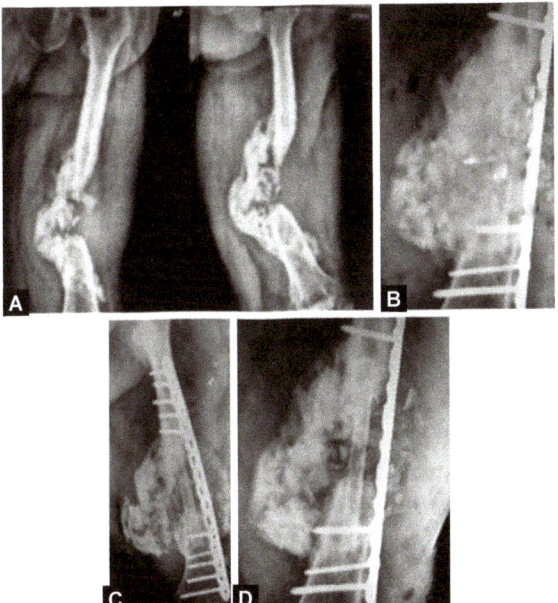

Figs. 10.24A to D: (A) Nonunion; (B to D) Treated with intramedullary fibula, long distal femur plate and massive cancellous bone graft.

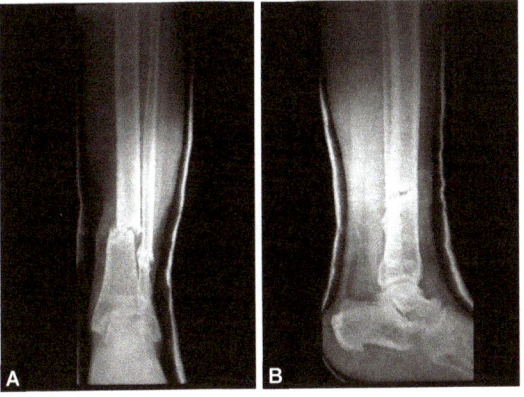

Figs. 10.25A and B: This 63-year-old patient was treated conservatively. (A) A.P.; (B) Lateral views.

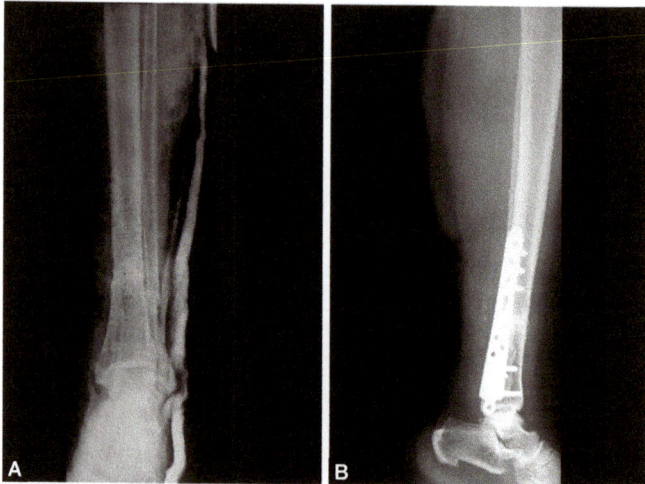

Figs. 10.26A and B: 63-years-old patient, fracture conserved for 5 months, nonunion.

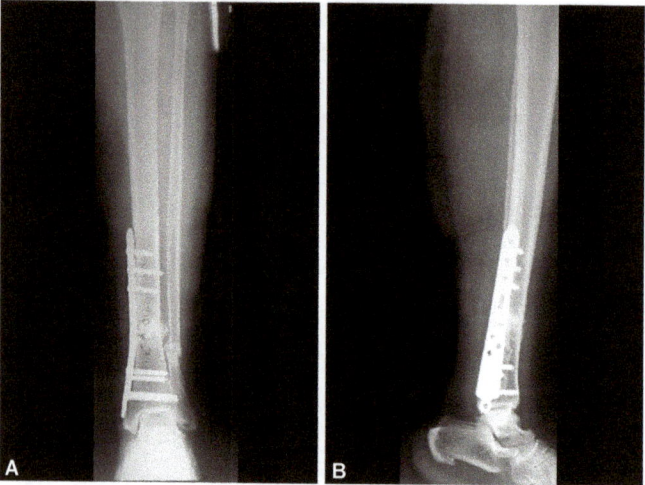

Figs. 10.27A and B: First surgery after failure of conservative. (A.P. and lateral views).

Chapter 10: Intramedullary Fibula for Treatment of Nonunion...

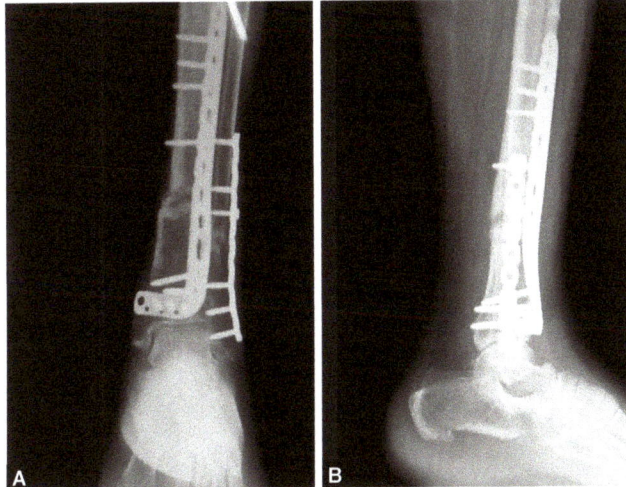

Figs. 10.28A and B: Failed second surgery. (A.P. and lateral views).

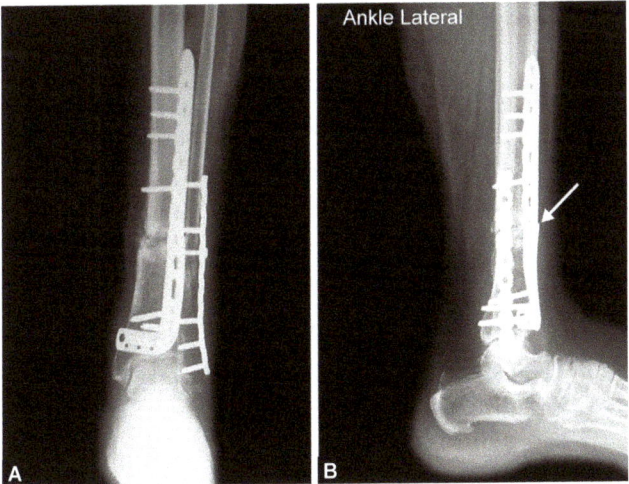

Figs. 10.29A and B: Failed second surgery, plate broken. (A.P. and lateral views).

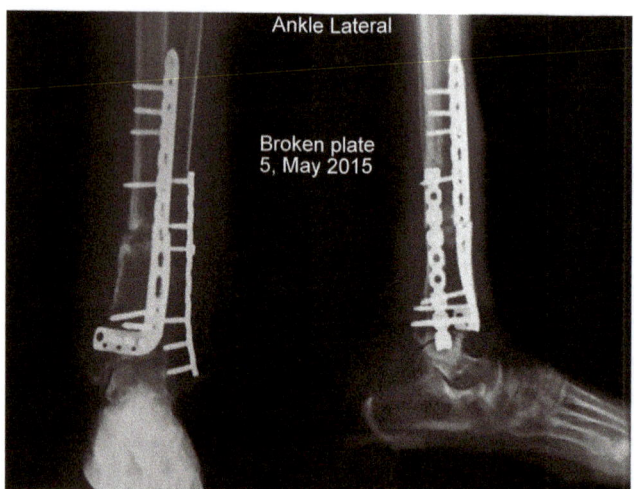

Fig. 10.30: Nonunion evident with implant failure.

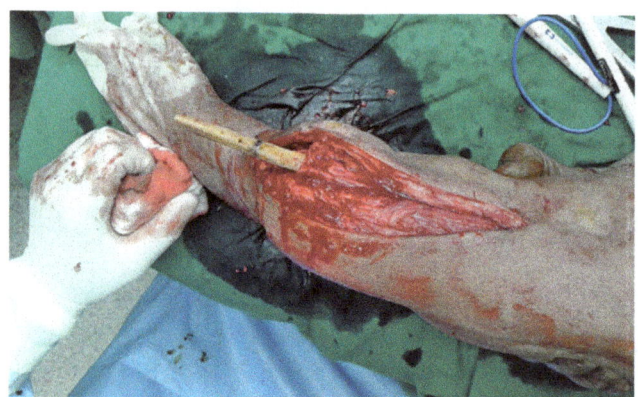

Fig. 10.31A: Intraoperative image with intramedullary fibula.

Chapter 10: Intramedullary Fibula for Treatment of Nonunion... 153

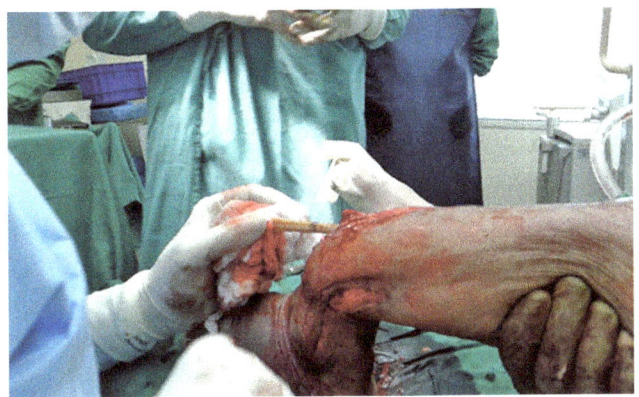

Fig. 10.31B: The fibula graft should move freely inside the medullary canal.

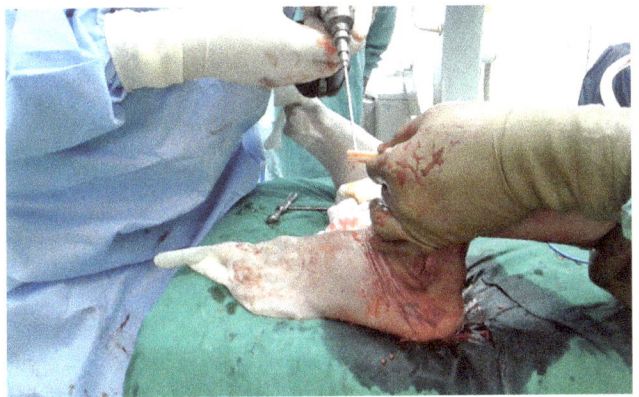

Fig. 10.32: Drill holes in fibula to propel inside.

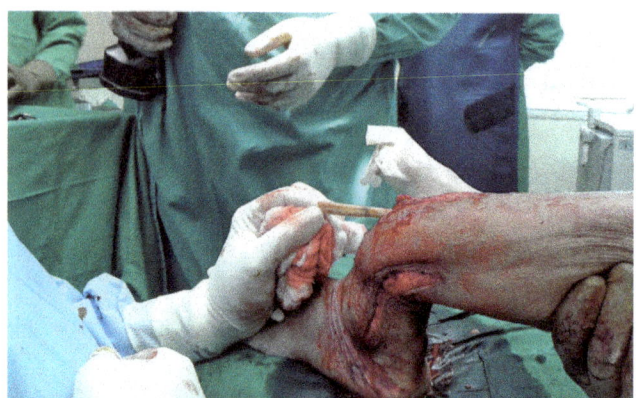

Fig. 10.33: Checking for smooth passage of the graft inside the canal.

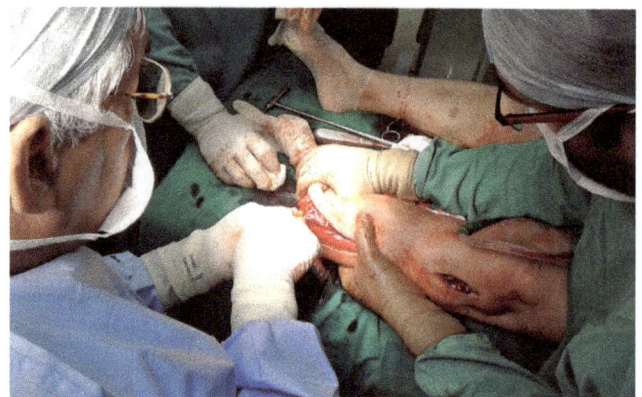

Fig. 10.34: Fibula graft pushed intramedullary.

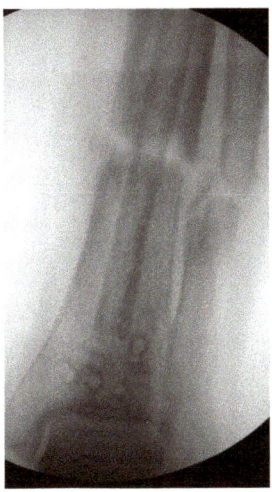

Fig. 10.35: Intraoperative.

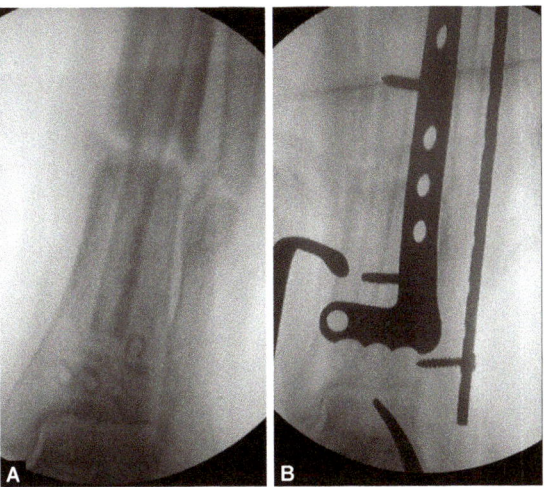

Figs. 10.36A and B: Intraoperative. (A) intramedullary fibula; (B) intramedullary fibula with plate.

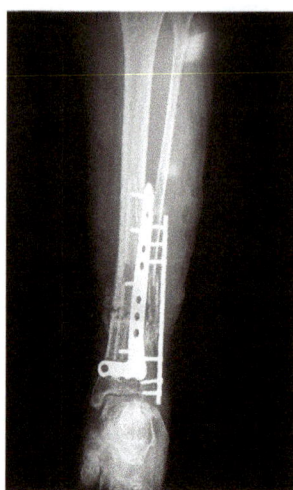

Fig. 10.37: Postoperative.

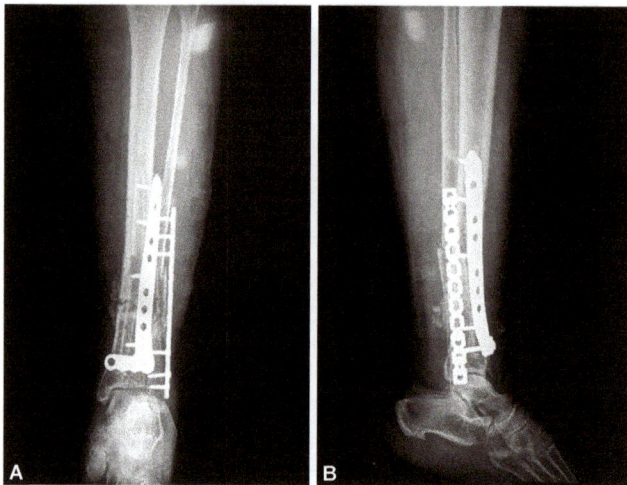

Figs. 10.38A and B: Follow-up X-ray images. (A.P. and lateral images).

Chapter 10: Intramedullary Fibula for Treatment of Nonunion...

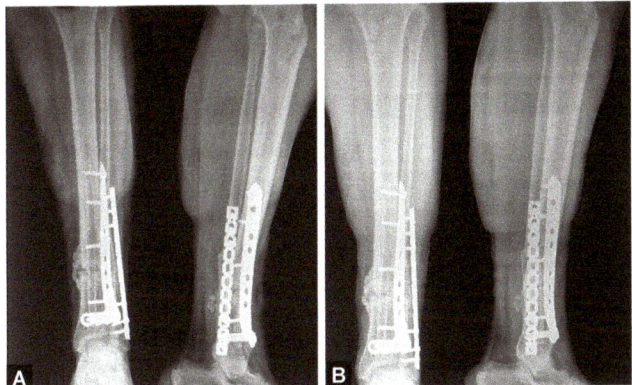

Figs. 10.39A and B: Subsequent follow-up X-ray images. (A.P. and lateral images).

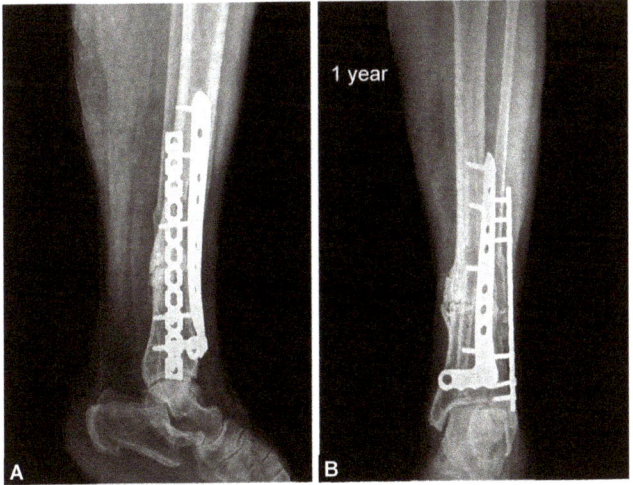

Figs. 10.40A and B: Slow healing at 1 year. (A.P. and lateral images).

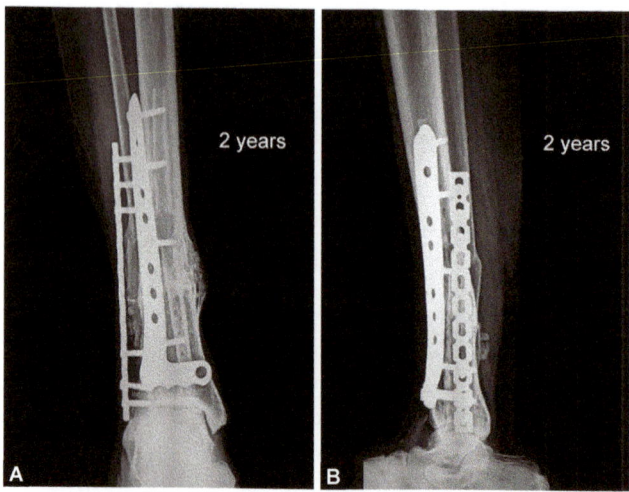

Figs. 10.41A and B: 2 year follow-up showing healing of fracture. (A.P. and lateral images).

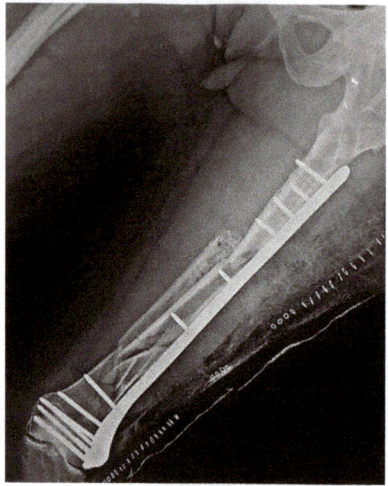

Fig. 10.42: First surgery, went into nonunion.

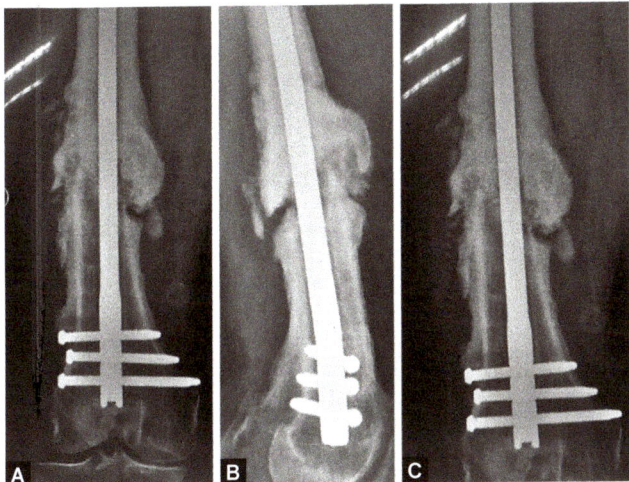

Figs. 10.43A to C: Second surgery.

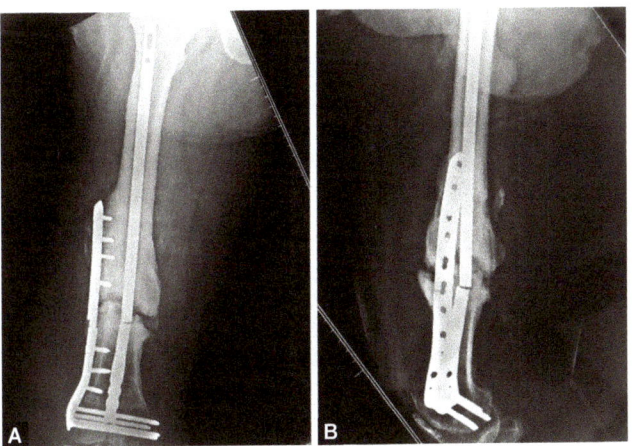

Figs. 10.44A and B: Broken nail with nonunion, surgeon could not remove nail. Added plate and graft. (A.P. and lateral images).

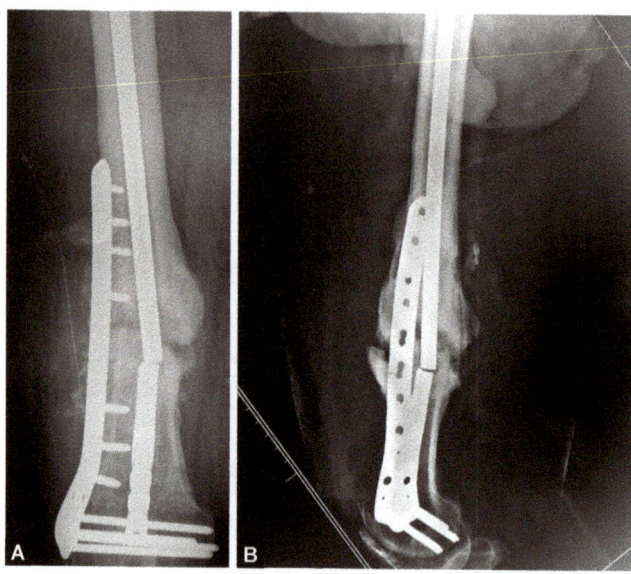

Figs. 10.45A and B: As expected nonunion.

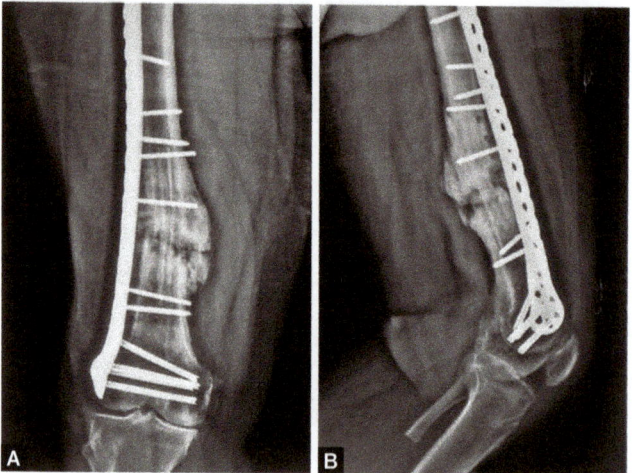

Figs. 10.46A and B: All implants removed, intramedullary fibula graft, medial cancellous graft and plate. (A.P. and lateral views).

Chapter 10: Intramedullary Fibula for Treatment of Nonunion...

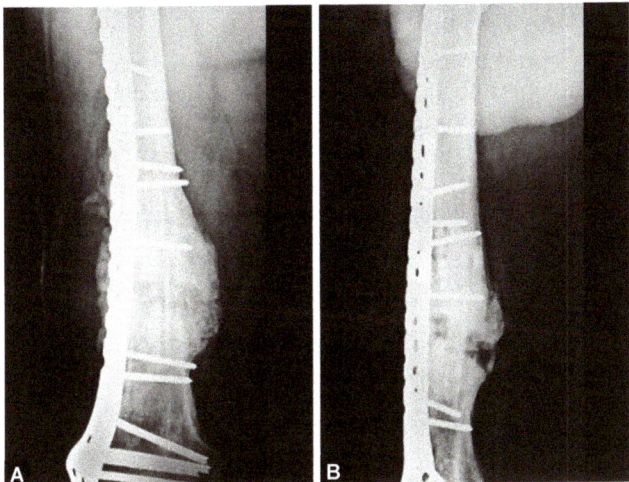

Figs. 10.47A and B: 9 months after surgery. (A.P. and lateral views).

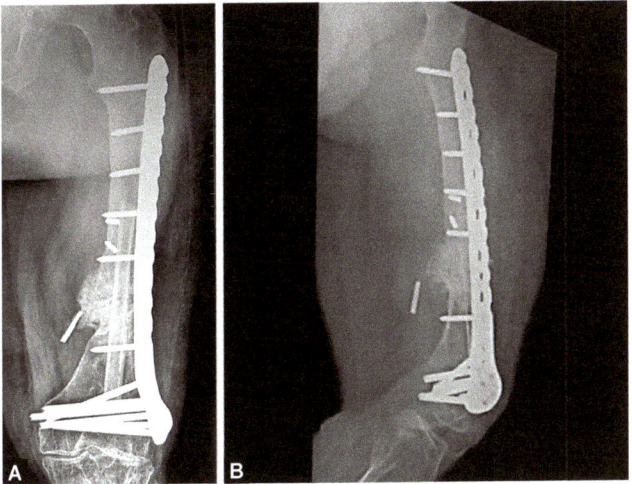

Figs. 10.48A and B: 1 year after surgery shows fracture healing. (A.P. and lateral views).

COMPLICATIONS

In long bones nonunions had no problem, except for one occasion, where fibula while trimming with bone cutter cracked. Now I do only with power instruments. Fibula in head of the femur for avascular necrosis (AVN) or fracture of neck femur. I have collected two cases where it penetrated the head of the femur and where total hip replacement (THR) was needed (Figs. 10.49 to 10.58).

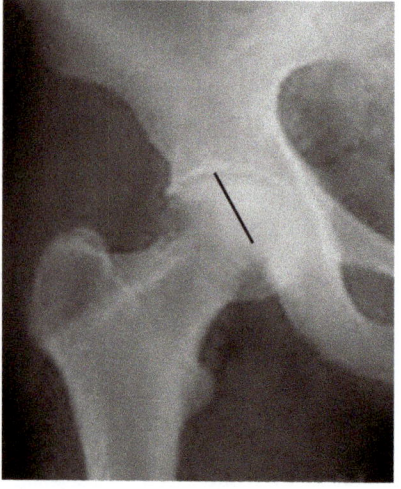

Fig. 10.49: Avascular necrosis (AVN) treated with intramedullary fibula. 28 years follow-up doing very well.

Chapter 10: Intramedullary Fibula for Treatment of Nonunion…

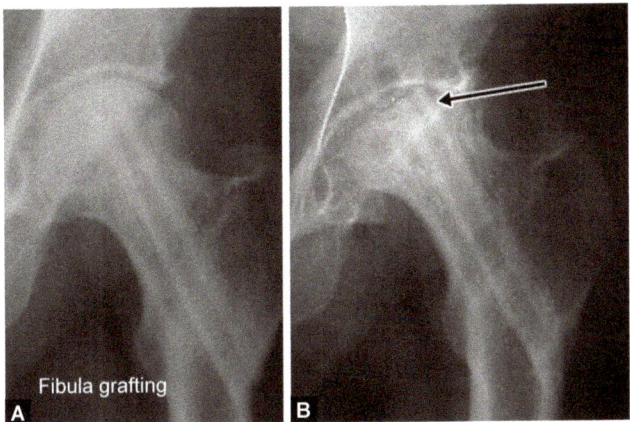

Figs. 10.50A and B: (A) Avascular necrosis (AVN) fibula intrafemoral; (B) Head collapsed, fibula goes in joint.

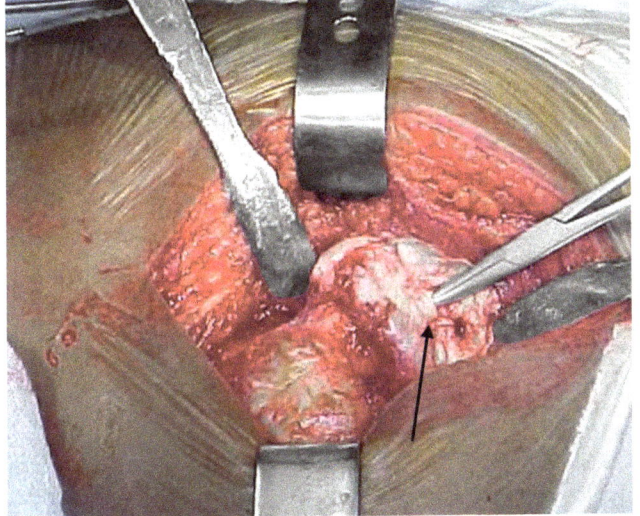

Fig. 10.51: While doing total hip replacement (THR) fibula seen penetrating the femur head.

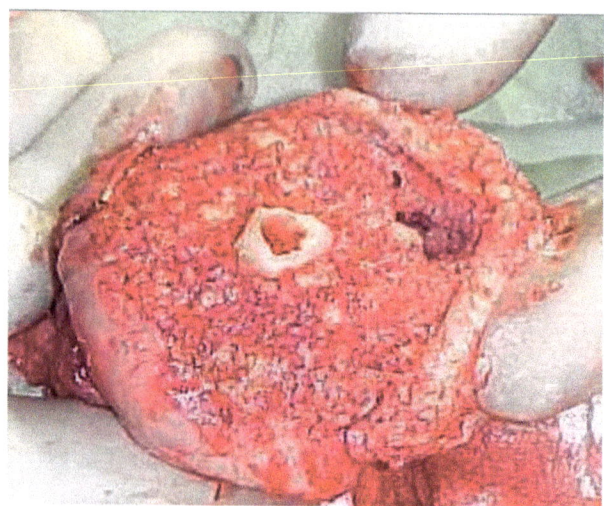

Fig. 10.52: While doing total hip replacement (THR) fibula seen penetrating the femur head.

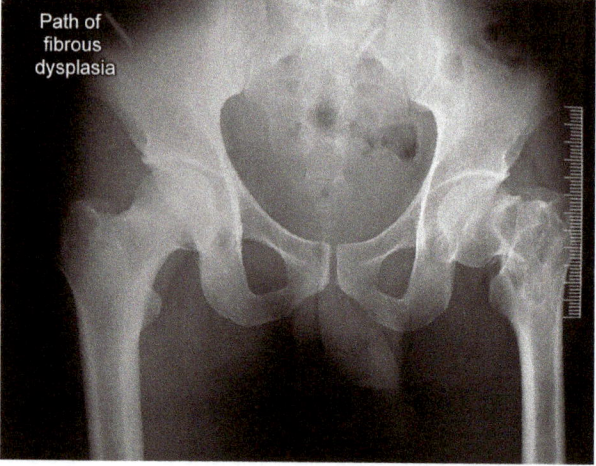

Fig. 10.53: Pathological fracture—Fibrous dysplasia of proximal femur.

Chapter 10: Intramedullary Fibula for Treatment of Nonunion...

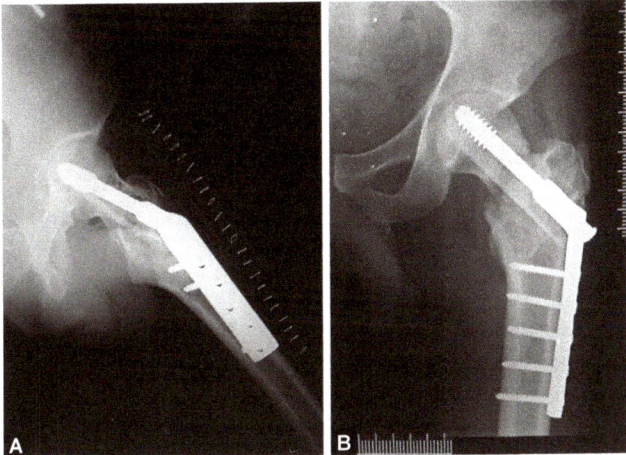

Figs. 10.54A and B: Dynamic hip screw (DHS) and fibula distally.

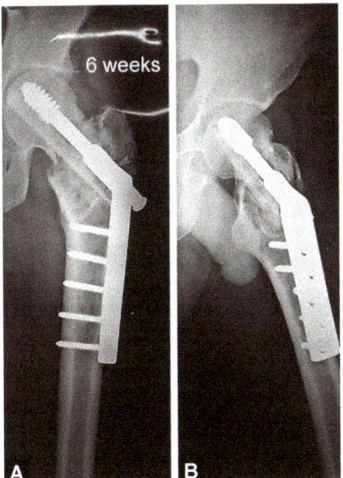

Figs. 10.55A and B: 6 weeks follow-up X-ray shows collapse. (A.P. and lateral views).

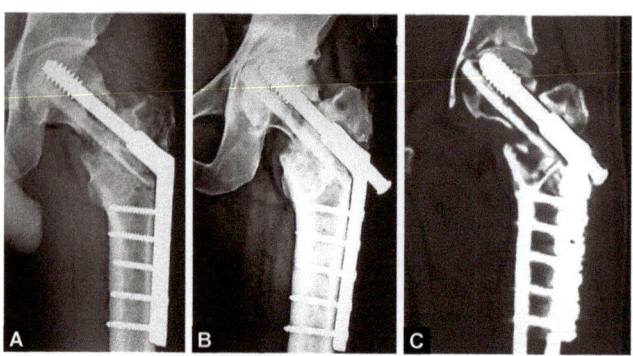

Figs. 10.56A to C: Fibula inside the joint after collapse on follow-up X-rays.

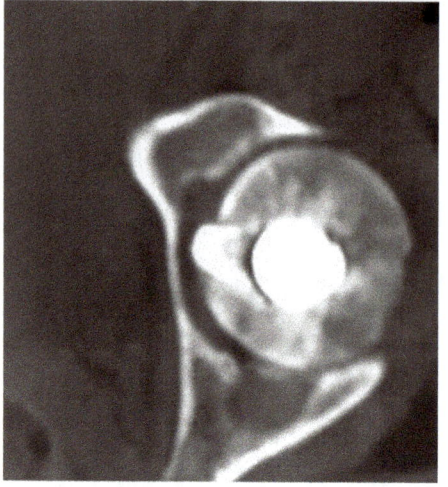

Fig. 10.57: CT confirms fibula inside the head and joint.

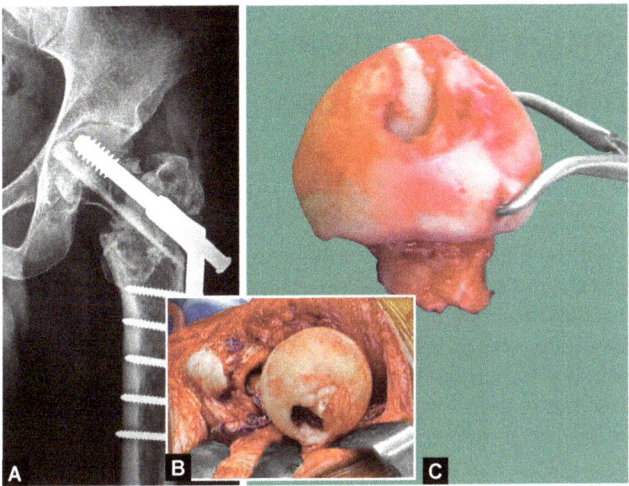

Figs. 10.58A to C: While doing total hip replacement (THR) fibula inside the joint. (A) X-ray; (B and C) Intraoperative images.

Syndesmotic Injury and Ankle Fracture

Chapter 11

DD Tanna

These three ligaments control the stability of syndesmotic joint. Medial ligament indirectly take part in stability of the syndesmotic joint. Interosseous membrane, if it is torn along with medial collateral ligament, will give syndesmotic instability. But if any one of it is torn alone it will not be unstable (Figs. 11.1A and B). If any one of them is torn, syndesmotic joint is not dislocated. Movements were consistently greater in the sagittal plane than the coronal plane and we conclude that distal tibiofibular instability should be assessed in the sagittal plane (anteroposterior). These three ligaments, interosseous membrane, anterior tibiofibular

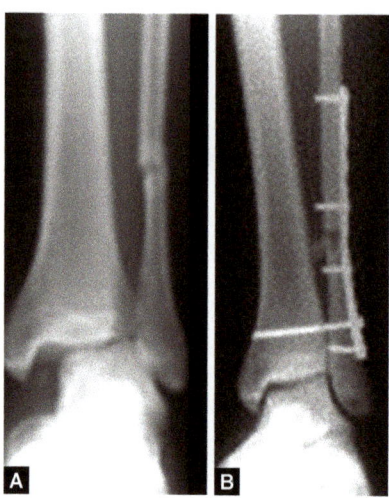

Figs. 11.1A and B: Typical syndesmotic injury.

Chapter 11: Syndesmotic Injury and Ankle Fracture

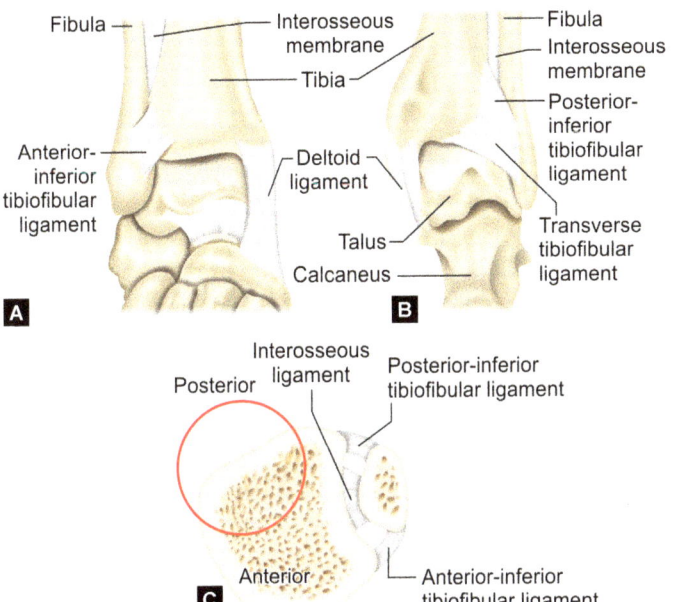

Figs. 11.2A to C: Three major ligamentous components provide stability to the syndesmosis, accounting for more than 90% of the total resistance to lateral fibular displacement.
(1) Anterior-inferior tibiofibular ligament; (2) Interosseous ligament; (3) Posterior-inferior tibiofibular ligament; (4) Medial, deltoid ligament, as additional.

ligament, posterior tibiofibular ligament control syndesmotic joint. Medial collateral ligament indirectly, takes part in stability of the syndesmotic joint, as mentioned earlier.

Abnormal movements were consistently greater in the sagittal plane than the coronal plane, if there is instability, of syndesmotic joint, so we conclude that distal tibiofibular instability should be assessed in the sagittal plane. Three ligaments control and stabilize the syndesmotic joint (Figs. 11.2A to C). Deltoid ligament adds to the stability along with interosseous membrane.

All these four ligaments which control the syndesmotic joint have a bone attached to it.

Ligamentous rupture and its bone attached
1. Anterior tibiofibular ligament > Tillaux fracture/chaput fracture
2. Posterior tibiofibular ligament > Posterior malleolus fracture
3. Interosseous ligament > Fracture fibula
4. Medial, deltoid ligament > Medial malleolus.

The ligament either rupture or bone attached with it fractures.

If all the four bones are fractured and we fix all four bones; we are re-establishing the syndesmotic ligament. And hence we do not need a syndesmotic screw.

When do we need syndesmotic screw?
When some ligaments are broken with bones, which we fix while other ligaments have no bony injury but ligaments have broken in substance. These ligaments need immobilization for healing, so fibula is fixed with tibia temporarily till ligaments heal (Fig. 11.3).

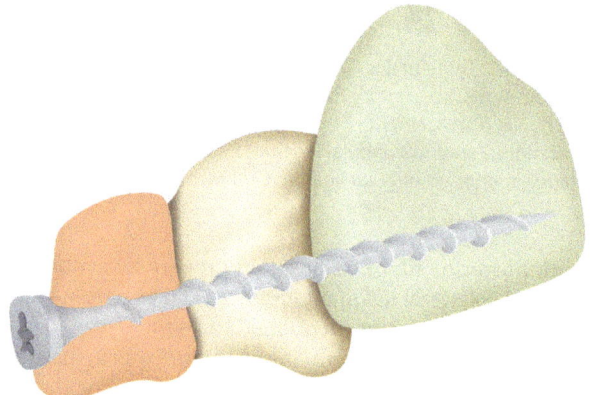

Fig. 11.3: Stitching the ligaments is not very fruitful. So we want them to heal in normal anatomy. Indirectly, keep fibula forcibly in its normal position so that ligaments will heal fully and reachieve stability which they had before injury.

So once bones are fixed, syndesmotic ligament is tested for stability by Cotton test (Fig. 11.4) for external and internal rotation of ankle. If stable, does not need any fixation of tibia to fibula and if unstable fibula is reduced by forward (Figs. 11.5 and 11.6) and internal rotation, and while it is reduced, it is temporarily fixed with K-wires posterior-to-anterior; and then in this reduced position, screws are put from fibula to tibia. Please observe that in syndesmotic injury, displacement of fibula is posteriorly and not laterally.

Now it is has been proved that two screws or one screw, 3–4 cm proximal and parallel to ankle joint, not in dorsiflexion but in neutral position is desirable. Three or four cortices, lag screw or position screw do not make difference. As ligaments take longer to heal, these screws are kept for 12–16 weeks till healing of ligaments occur and not removed after 6 weeks as believed

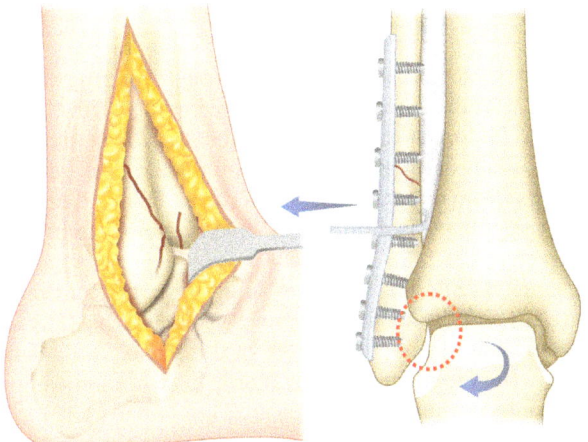

Fig. 11.4: Standard practice of syndesmotic injury fixations. Reduce medial malleolus, reduce lateral malleolus. Judge if posterior malleolus needs repair. Do Cotton test if needed, put two syndesmotic screws biting three cortices.

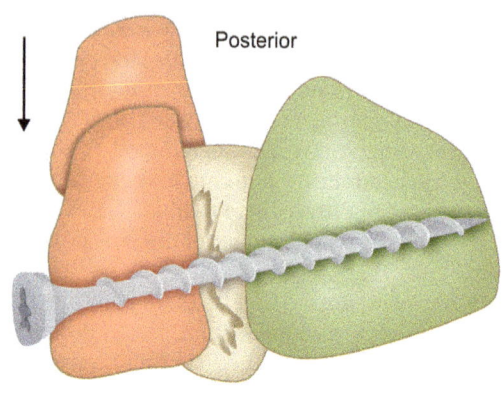

Fig. 11.5: Fibula is reduced by forward and internal rotation fixed temporarily with K-wires in posterior-anterior direction. Fix definitely with two tricortical screws in the same direction.

earlier. These screws may break on weight bearing which is started in 6 weeks' time without removing the screws as they are needed for longer time. On weight bearing, these screws can break, so if four cortices are engaged, broken part of screw can be removed from opposite side of the cortex. To avoid this screw breakage, tightrope is introduced, which is now recommended (Figs. 11.7A to C).

If screw is catching 3 cortices it l loosen and not break on walking, if 4 cortices are fixed. It can break on walking (Fig. 11.8).

It has been observed that 33% of the times, fibula is fixed without perfect reduction, which is only detected in postoperative computed tomography (CT) scan (Figs. 11.9 to 11.12).

In order to avoid this malreduction, it is recommended that after reduction and temporary K-wire fixation and before putting screws or tightrope, open the syndesmotic joint anteriorly and

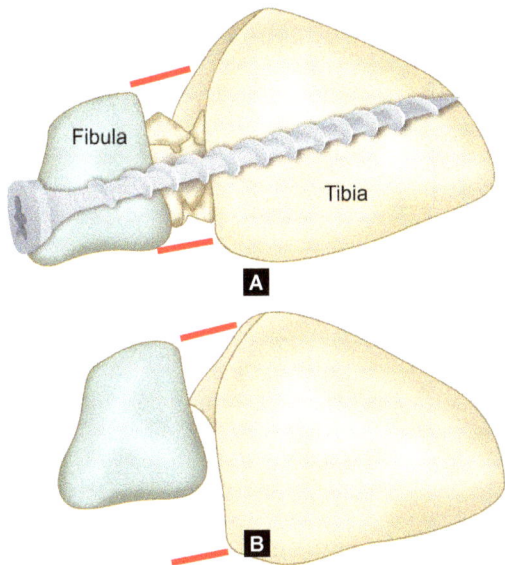

Figs. 11.6A and B: (A) When properly reduced and screw put in, ligaments heal properly; (B) When syndesmotic joint is not reduced properly and fixed, ligaments do not heal and joint is unstable.

confirm that it is reduced properly (Figs. 11.13 and 11.14). See Mercedes-Benz sign for reduction.

If posterior malleolus is not fixed, fibula tends to displace posteriorly. So fixing of posterior malleolus is necessary to reduce joint (Fig. 11.15).

Recognition of a problem is easy because the talus is subluxated in the same direction as the fibula is displaced (Fig. 11.16).

Concepts of syndesmotic injury have changed. We must follow the newer understanding.

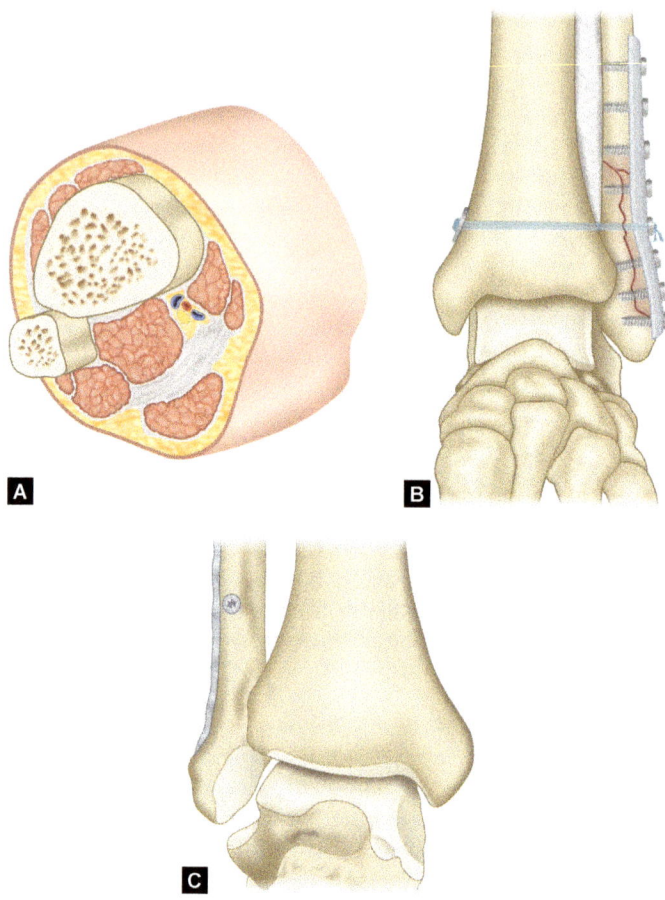

Figs. 11.7A to C: Tightrope fixation: This tightrope is currently popular.

Chapter 11: Syndesmotic Injury and Ankle Fracture

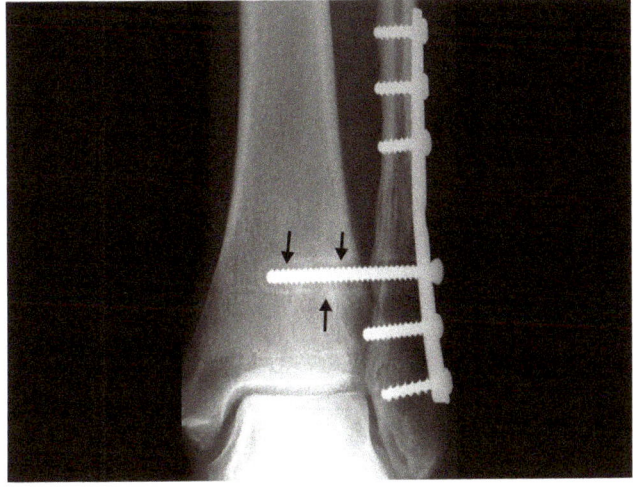

Fig. 11.8: Three cortices it will loosen not break.

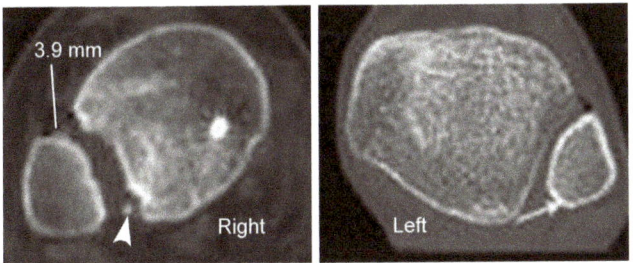

Fig. 11.9: Postoperative CT shows displaced joint on right compared to left.

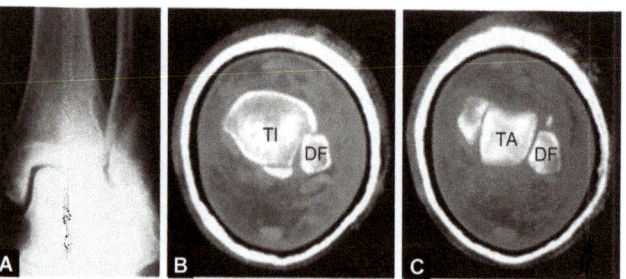

Figs. 11.10A to C: Postoperative CT detects 33% of reductions are defective.

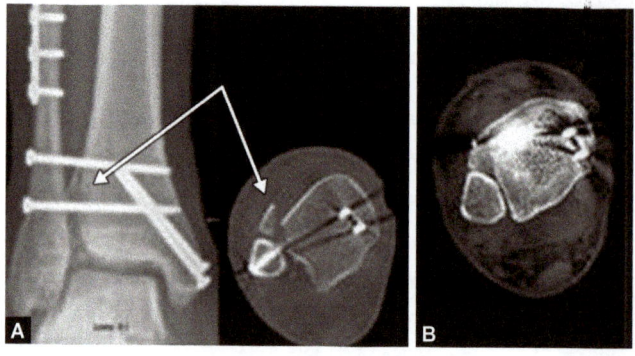

Figs. 11.11A and B: Postoperative CT reveals 33% of the time, syndesmosis is not well reduced on postoperative CT scan.

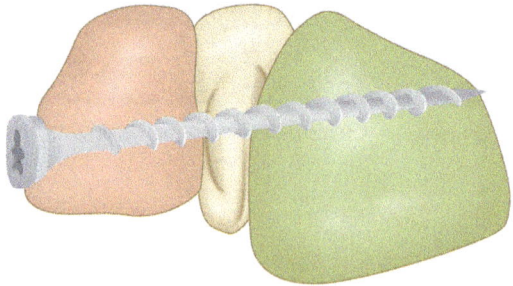

Fig. 11.12: Often it happens that joint is fixed with inadequate reduction.

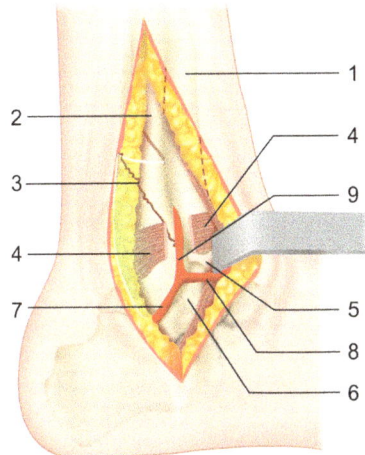

Fig. 11.13: Open syndesmotic joint and see this Mercedes-Benz sign to confirm perfect reduction.

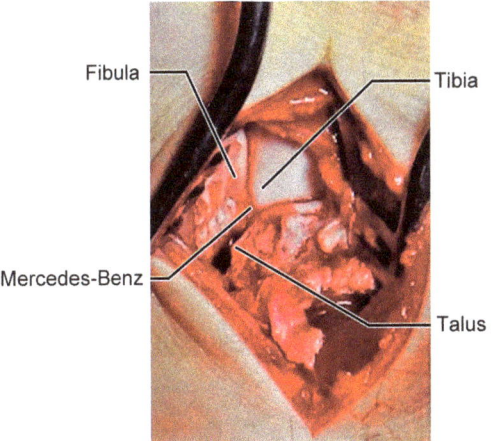

Fig. 11.14: Vision when we open the joint to confirm reduction.

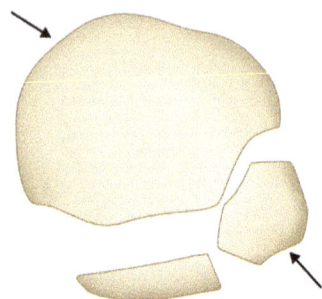

Fig. 11.15: If posterior malleolus is not fixed, fibula tends to displace posteriorly, so fixing of posterior malleolus is necessary to reduce joint.

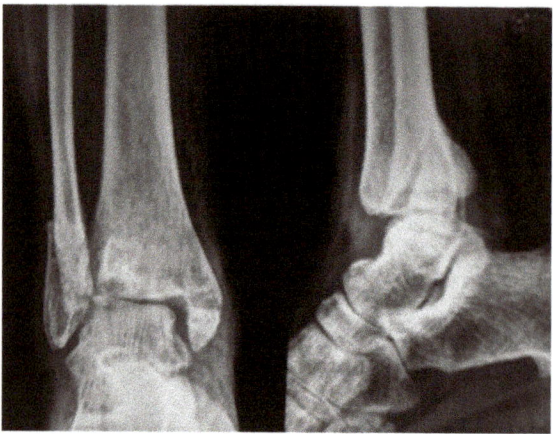

Fig. 11.16: Recognition of problem is easy because the talus is subluxated in the same direction as the fibula is displaced.

Chapter 12

Posterior Malleolus

DD Tanna

Practice of fixing posterior malleolus from anteroposterior blindly, is now no more valid.

Not fixing posterior malleolus which is 15–20% is also debated. Computed tomography (CT) scan is a must to assess posterior malleolus (Figs. 12.1A to D). Posterior malleolus, when fractured has attachment of posterior tibiofibular ligament.

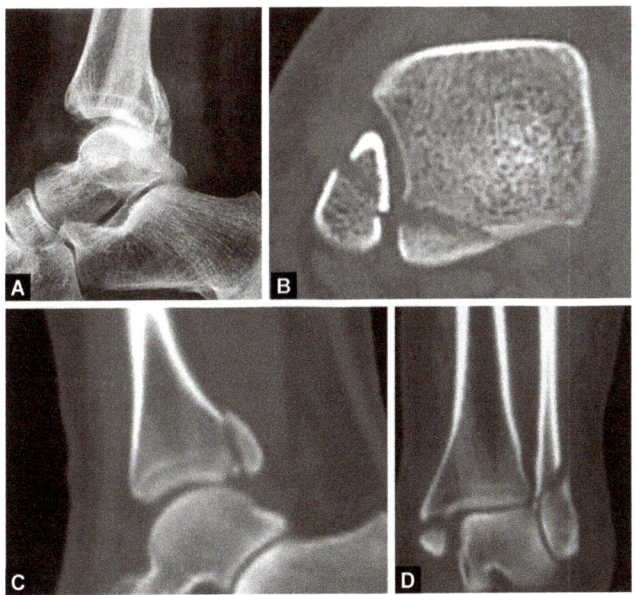

Figs. 12.1A to D: I do not treat ankle fracture without CT scan as posterior malleolus is missed and type of posterior malleolus is not clear for fixation.

So fixation of all posterior malleolus is needed to re-establish integrity of this ligament (Figs. 12.2A to C).

Since fracture can be a small piece at an angle on lateral side or complete posterior part of tibia, it needs identification and

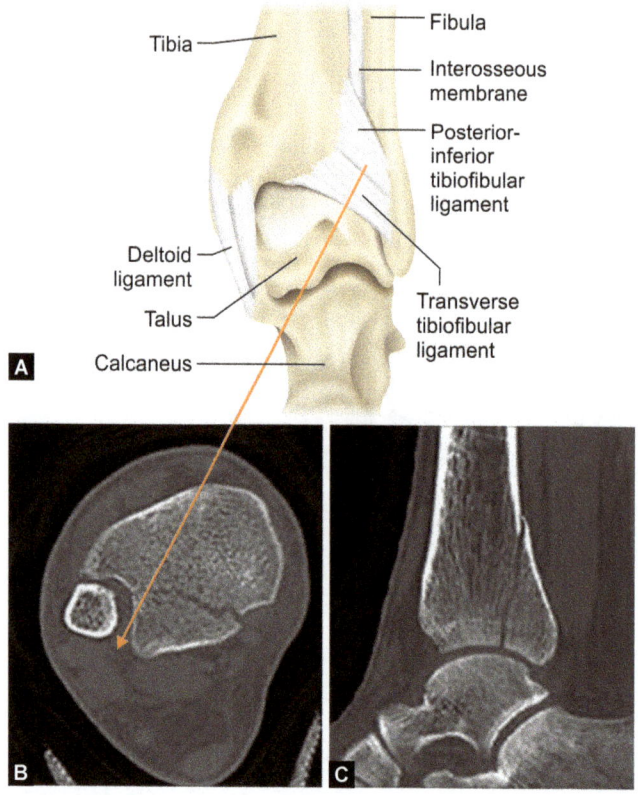

Figs. 12.2A to C: It is important to understand that the posterior malleolus is where the posterior-inferior tibiofibular ligament (PITFL) attaches and this ligament imparts most of the stability to the syndesmotic region and thus to the ankle joint. Posterior malleolus is not bone fixation, it is fixation of PITFL. So fix posterior malleolus, even if small, to fix the strong ligament.

that can be done only with CT scan, so CT is must to know where posterior malleolus is fractured. Posterior malleolus needs either a lag screw or buttress plate. Most of the time, post-incision will address both plating of fibula and screw or buttress plate for posterior malleolus.

Posterior malleolus needs fixation, if displaced, small or large, it should be fixed from posterior-anterior and *not anterior-posterior* (Figs. 12.3 to 12.6). This is a special type of a fracture

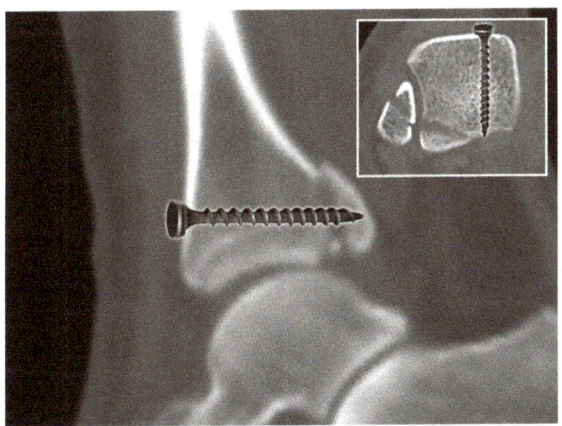

Fig. 12.3: I do not do anterior-posterior fixation of posterior malleolus as it may not bite fracture fragment as shown.

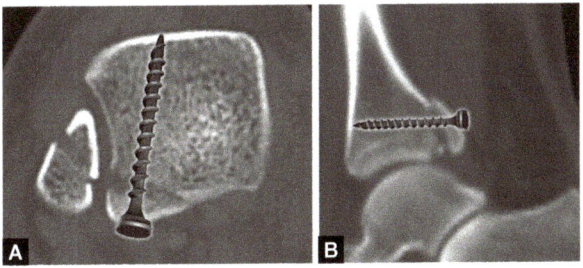

Figs. 12.4A and B: Put screw from posterior-anterior. Then one can fix from the center of such fragment and get compression of the fracture.

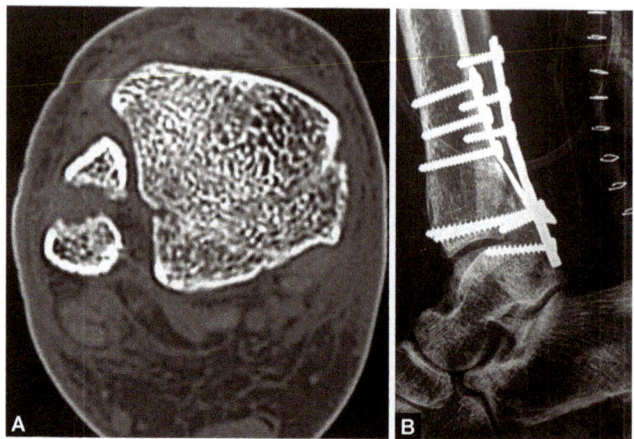

Figs. 12.5A and B: Computed tomography (CT) if shows such large piece of posterior malleolus, it will need buttress plate from posterior. At times as the fragment is large, we will need two buttress plates.

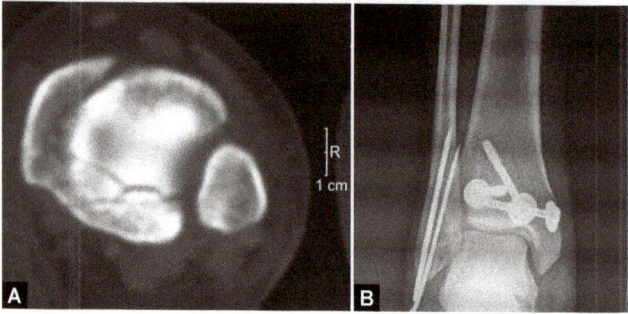

Figs. 12.6A and B: This is a special type of a fracture where posterior fracture and medial fracture is considered, one piece fracture, unless the fracture is reduced simultaneously from posterior and medial, it will not reduce. If one fixes posterior malleolus or medial malleolus separately, it will not reduce.

where posterior fracture and medial fracture is considered, one piece fracture, unless the fracture is reduced simultaneously from posterior and medial, it will not reduce. If one fixes posterior malleolus or medial malleolus separately, it will not reduce.

Elbow Dislocation with Irreparable Fracture of Head of Radius

Chapter 13

DD Tanna

Elbow dislocation is very inadequately treated due to confusions of ideas. Elbow dislocation without any associated fracture needs no special care except reduction if needed under sedation or short anesthesia and splint for few days till pain subsides, and then rehabilitation. Those dislocations with associated fractures of head of radius need repair of head of radius or replacement of the head of radius with reduction of dislocation to achieve a stable reduction. Results of repair or replacement of radial head are not always satisfactory for supination pronation movements though elbow remains stable.

Now the question that comes to mind is why excision of *isolated fracture of head of radius* gives very satisfactory results, except few reports of proximal migration of radius over years? While excision of head of radius in elbow dislocation gives unsatisfactory results due to elbow instability.

Elbow dislocation, with irreparable fracture of head of radius, needs replacement of the head of radius to achieve stable elbow. If head of radius is repairable, it must be repaired.

Normal day-to-day isolated, irreparable head of radius fracture can be treated with excision of head of radius with very little or no major problem because medial collateral ligament (MCL) is intact unlike in elbow dislocation. Before excising this head of radius, under anesthesia, it must be confirmed that there is no instability and this radius fracture is not a part of original elbow dislocation which has been reduced outside or autoreduced.

In elbow dislocation, MCL is always injured. If excision of head of radius is done for irreparable head of radius fracture, there is increased chance of redislocation. This head of radius must be replaced with artificial radial head prosthesis. Results of replacement of head of radius are also not consistent, there are many long-term and short-term failures. Design of the head of radius is also not consistent.

I felt that when MCL is not injured in isolated fracture of the head of radius, head excision gives consistent results. Then in elbow dislocation, if radial head is not repairable and needs replacement, why not excise head of radius and re-establish medial collateral integrity.

I started doing in such cases, excision of head of radius and repair of MCL and was happy to have good results. Now even though radial head replacement implants are available, I feel this is a decent option to consider.

The method I followed, is on arrival elbow dislocation was confirmed on plain X-ray, and elbow was reduced under sedation in all cases except in one where because of apprehension, short general anesthesia was used.

After reduction, X-ray image was taken in anteroposterior (AP) and lateral view to exactly assess the pattern of associated fracture. Computed tomography (CT) scan was done in few cases as it was felt that it was not necessary in all cases. Those cases with associated fracture of the repairable radial head were repaired and were immobilized with plaster for 2 weeks. Those radial heads which were not repairable and needed replacement were the only ones which were the subject of the discussion. In all such cases, radial head was excised as it was irreparable or I could not repair them due to lack of small implants and/or lack of necessary skills. I could not think of replacing them as implants were not available in India at that time.

I exposed the joint from mid-line posterior approach on either side of the triceps. Head of radius was observed and when found irreparable, I excised it. MCL was exposed and it was observed that it was completely torn along with medial origin of the muscles in a few of my cases.

Medial collateral ligament was sutured with thick, nonabsorbable Ethibond sutures, and medial stability was established. It should be remembered that out of the two bands, the anterior band of the MCL is most important and essential to be sutured. Muscles which were torn, also were sutured. I had not used anchors on medial side. At the end of the procedure, stability of the elbow was checked. If coronoid piece was avulsed, it was sutured with pull-through sutures. Small piece of coronoid was neglected. If coronoid needs repair, it must be done before collateral suturing as it is seen in the wound very easily when medial collateral is not yet sutured. At the end of the procedure when stability was satisfactory, wound was closed, and above elbow plaster was given for 6 weeks for soft tissue healing (Figs. 13.1 to 13.10).

After removal of plaster, slow increasing range of movements, and muscle strengthening exercises were done and good range of movements were obtained in all cases. All patients were seen till 4 months after removal of plaster, and were assessed for range of movements and elbow stability. All elbows were stable. None had any problem with day-to-day activity. None were sports people.

During my early days, there was non-availability of head of radius prosthesis. I was treating elbow dislocations with radial head fractures by keeping shattered radial head intact and immobilizing the elbow with temporary strong Steinmann

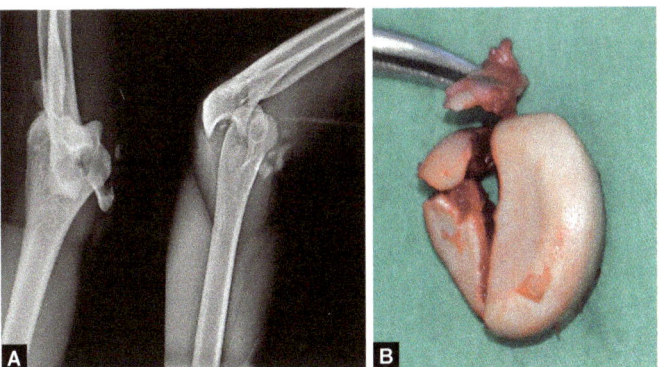

Figs. 13.1A and B: Dislocation of elbow with irreparable fracture of head of radius.

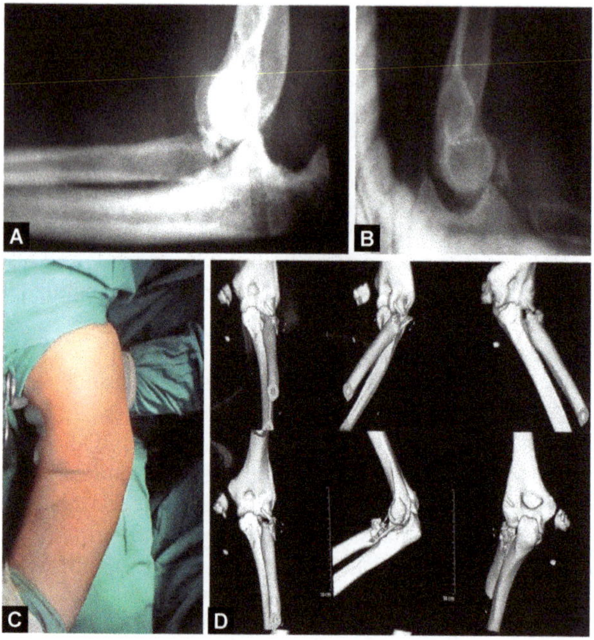

186 *Orthopedic Secrets*

Figs. 13.2A to D: X-ray and computed tomography scan.

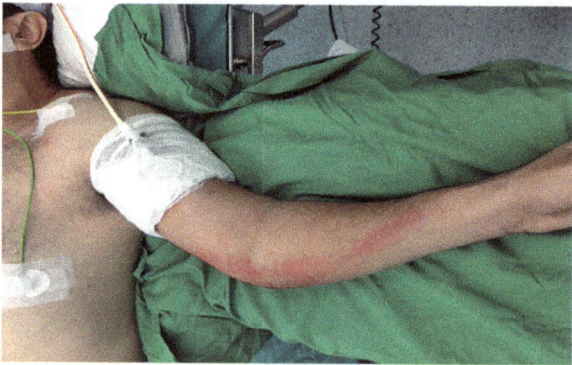

Fig. 13.3: Preoperative.

Chapter 13: Elbow Dislocation with Irreparable Fracture of ...

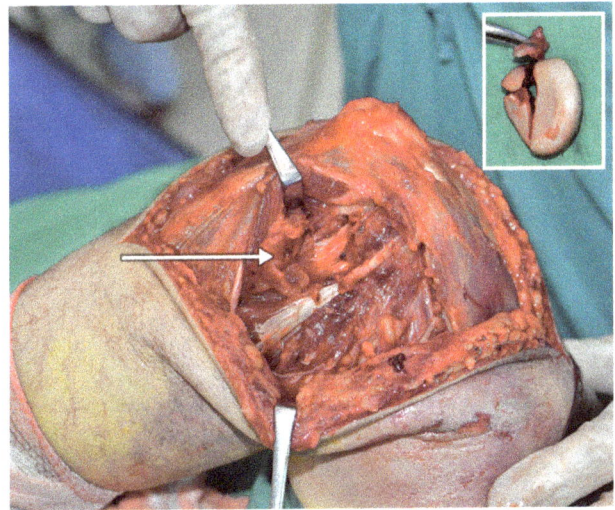

Fig. 13.4: Avulsion, medial group of muscles with medial collateral ligament and excised radial head in corner.

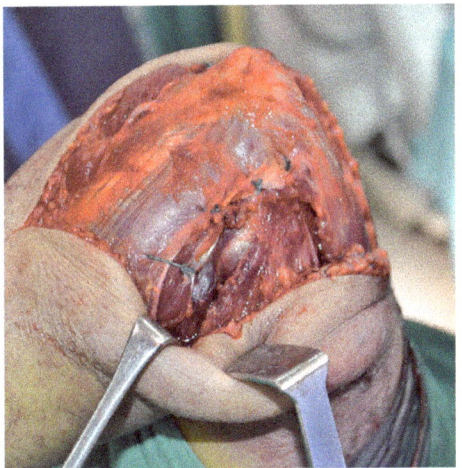

Fig. 13.5: Sutured medial collateral ligament and medial muscle.

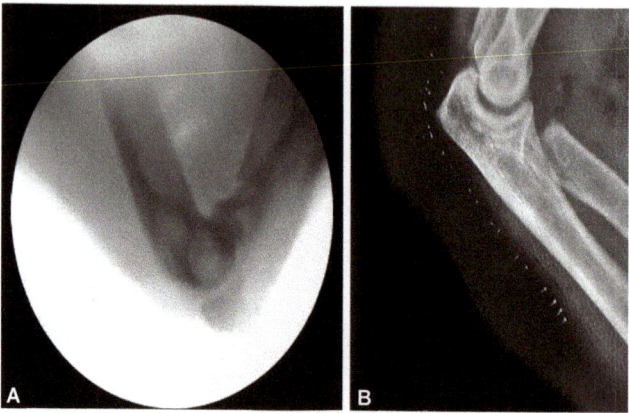

Figs. 13.6A and B: Intraoperative test for stability and final X-ray.

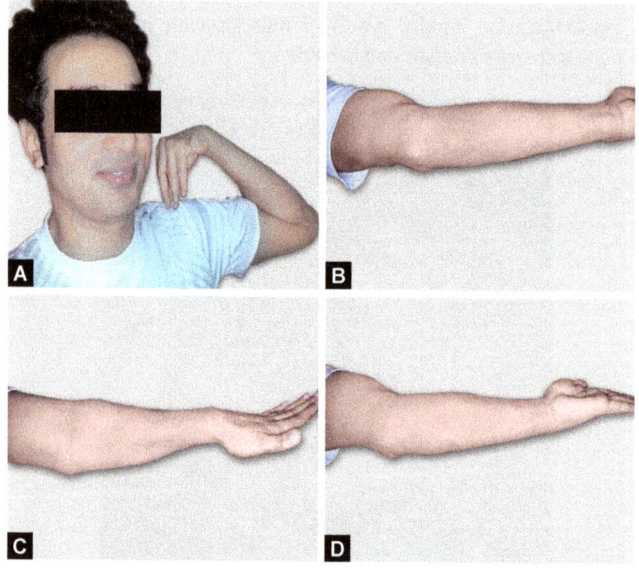

Figs. 13.7A to D: Clinical movements.

Chapter 13: Elbow Dislocation with Irreparable Fracture of ...

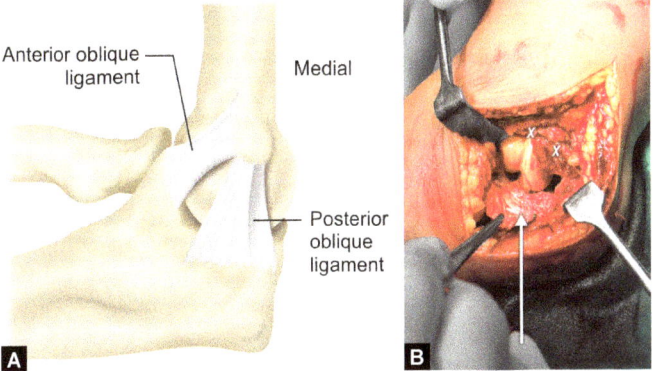

Figs. 13.8A and B: Important anterior medial collateral ligament band identified.

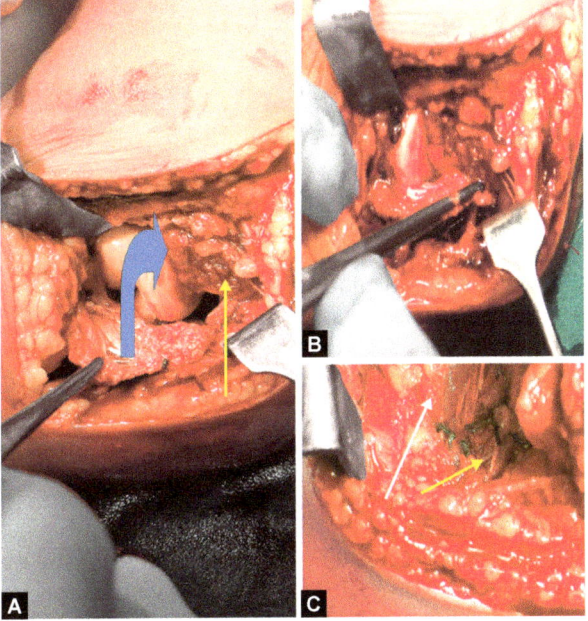

Figs. 13.9A to C: Medial collateral ligament sutured.

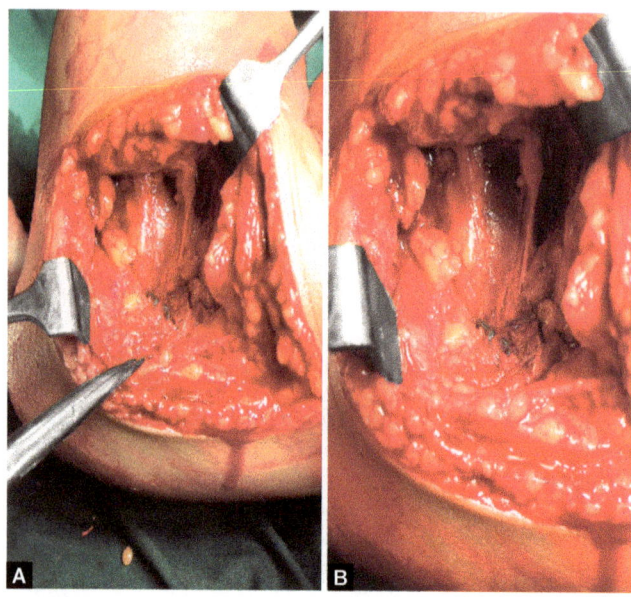

Figs. 13.10A and B: At the end of suturing.

pin from olecranon to humerus for 4 weeks. The comminuted head of radius was excised after about 2–3 months to regain supination pronation. Unfortunately, supination pronation did not return fully in these cases. Initially I was using strong K-wire to immobilize these elbows after reduction. I observed that these K-wires would bend and at times break giving lot of problems. I switched over to strong Steinmann pins.

Later on I started excising the radial head, primarily and forcibly keeping elbow reduced by Steinmann pin. I observed that elbow was not stable even after this, and had marked restriction of movements.

When I changed over this treatment to excising the radial head and repairing the MCL, I observed that elbows were stable and full movements were achieved even within 6 weeks of plaster.

Primary stabilizer of the elbow is intact bones, namely intact olecranon and coronoid, intact head of radius, and intact lower end of the humerus. Medial and lateral collateral ligaments are secondary stabilizers of the elbow.

Simple day-to-day irreparable fracture head of radius can be excised without any inferior result. This cannot be done with associated elbow dislocation, as if radial head is excised, both primary and secondary stabilizers are absent and hence elbow will redislocate even in plaster. So if any one stabilizer is intact, elbow is stable, like excised radial head in simple dislocation where MCL is intact, elbow is stable. In dislocation without suturing MCL, if irreparable head of radius is replaced, elbow is stable even with ruptured MCL. So you need only one stabilizer of elbow for stability.

And so I started excising the irreparable fracture head of radius and re-establishing secondary stabilizer by resuturing MCL and have found an excellent substitute to replacement in this treatment.

Basically, if I can, excise radial head without dislocation where MCL is intact, than, I can excise head and suture MCL, and that elbow will also be stable. Initial success encouraged me to continue this.

So in conclusion I feel this is a better approach in irreparable head of radius fracture with elbow dislocation, if one wants to avoid, replacement. Repair of head radius if possible must be done, without any doubt.

Reamer/Irrigator/Aspirator (RIA) System: Use with induced Membrane to Fill-up Bone Defects

Chapter 14

RM Chandak

The evolution of contemporary intramedullary reaming systems has recently generated the Reamer/Irrigator/Aspirator system (RIA-Synthes), which has progressively gained popularity, as it yields impressive volumes of the osteoinductive and osteogenic reamings for grafting purposes.

The RIA device is a single-pass reamer that is connected to an aspirator and irrigator through two separate ports permitting the surgeon to simultaneously ream, irrigate, and aspirate contents from the femoral canal, at the tip of the reamer. The harvested bone graft is then collected into a filtered suction cup that separates cancellous bone from the supernatant fluid. Following case is of a 30-year-old male who sustained road traffic accident. Complete follow-up of the case is presented in Figures 14.1 to 14.19.

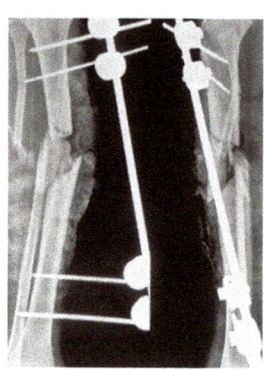

Fig. 14.1: A 30-year-old male sustained injury from road traffic accident and had compound fracture of tibia, fibula grade IIIB, with exposed bones; initially managed with external fixator.

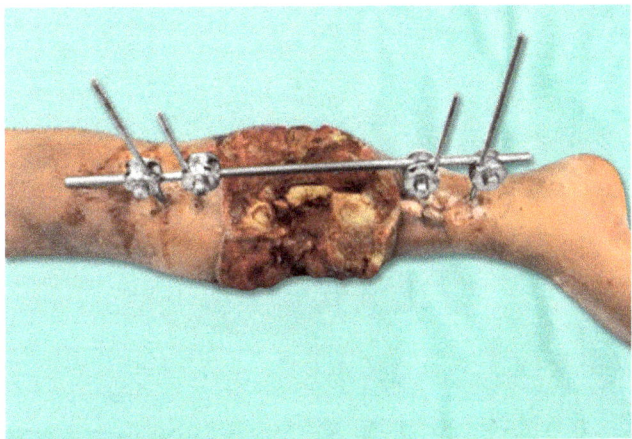

Fig. 14.2: Wound condition on presentation to our hospital 12 days after accident; infection, slough, and foul smell.

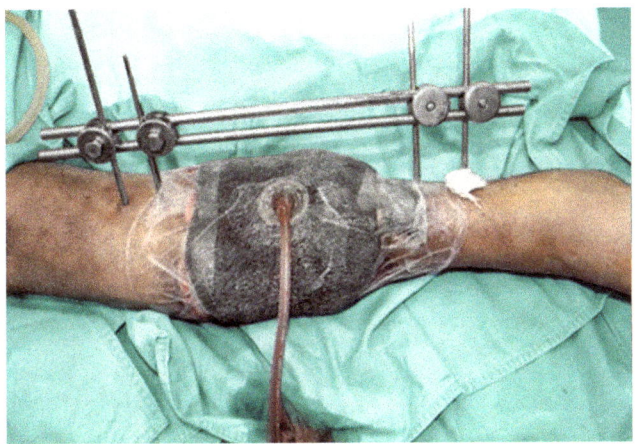

Fig. 14.3: Meticulous debridement—wash/lavage and vaccum assisted closure (VAC) application done.

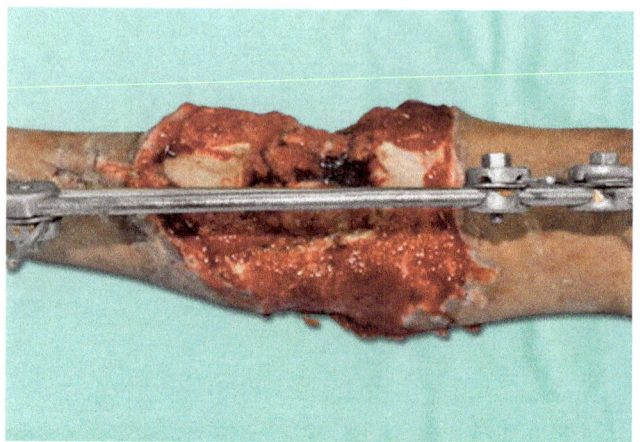

Fig. 14.4: After 1st vaccum assisted closure (VAC) dressing application, healthy bed of soft tissues.

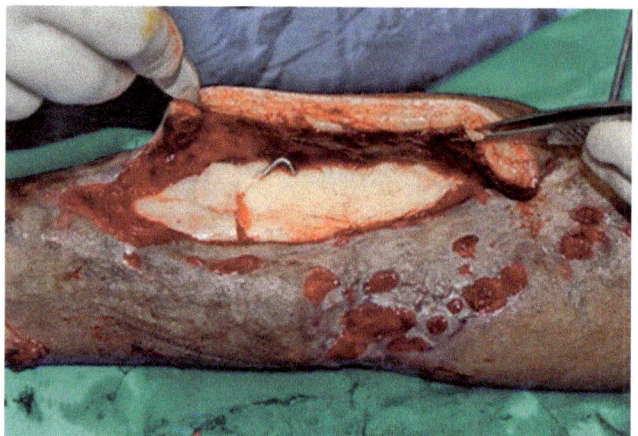

Fig. 14.5: Antibiotic cement spacer with 4 gm of vancomycin.

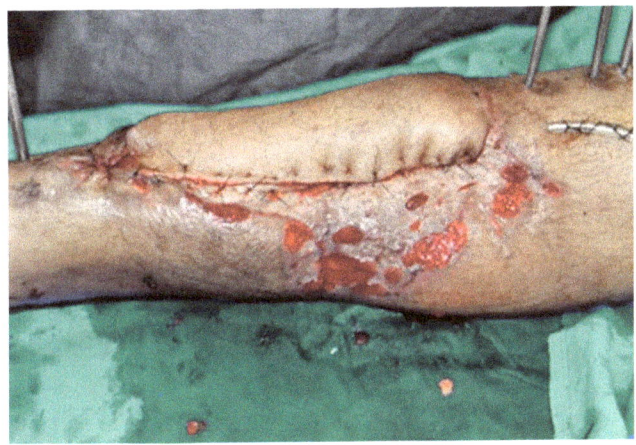

Fig. 14.6: Antibiotic spacer flap done and taken up well.

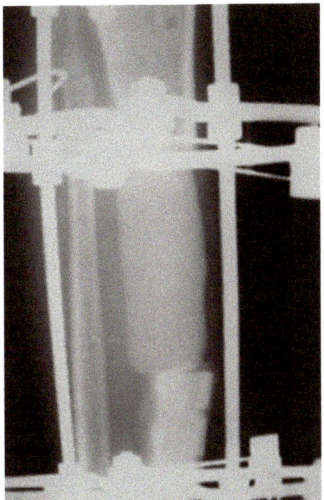

Fig. 14.7: Antibiotic bone cement block—planned for Reamer/Irrigator/Aspirator (RIA) grafts. Note the girth.

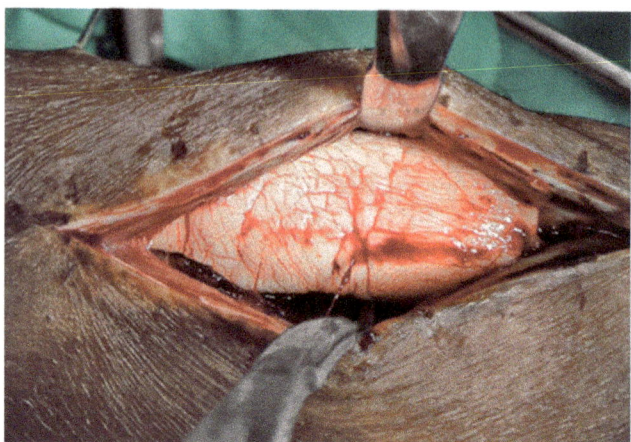

Fig. 14.8: Cement block prepares the periosteal tube with induced membrane.

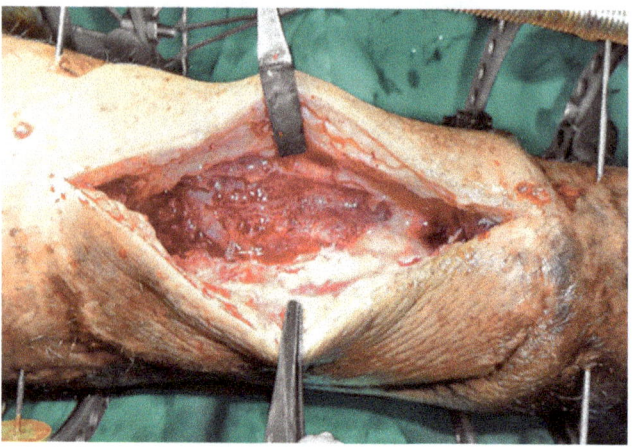

Fig. 14.9: This large 6-inch bone gap needs large volume of grafts after removal of antibiotic cement spacer.

Chapter 14: Reamer/Irrigator/Aspirator (RIA) System...

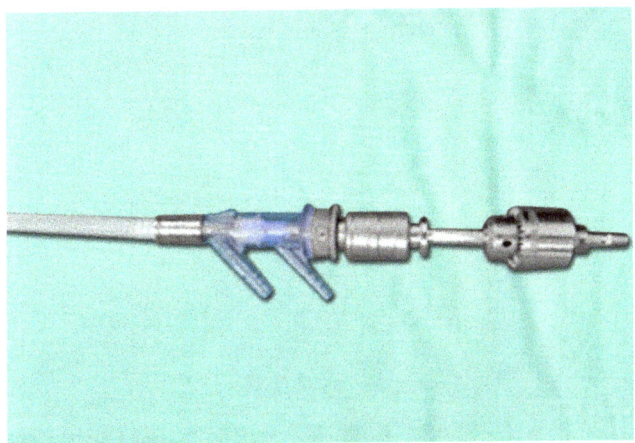

Fig. 14.10: Picture shows Reamer/Irrigator/Aspirator device mounted on drill chuck.

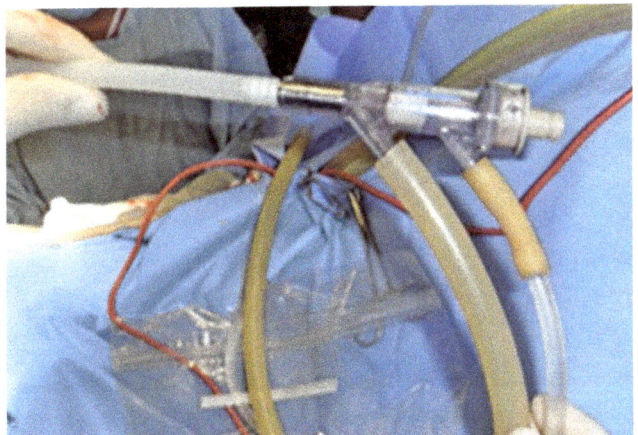

Fig. 14.11: Picture shows Reamer/Irrigator/Aspirator (RIA) tube assembly with connections for saline irrigation port and suction port (large tube for graft filter).

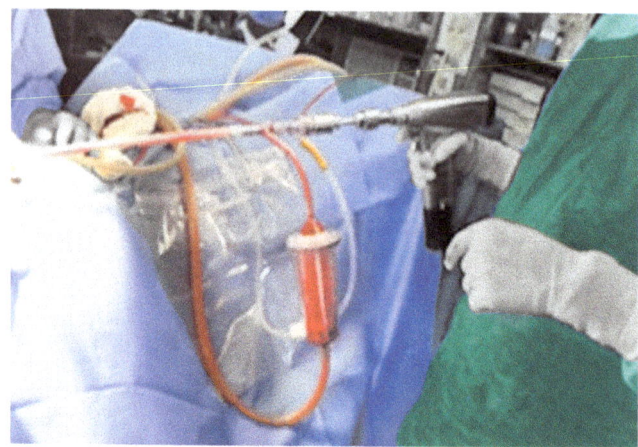

Fig. 14.12: Picture shows active process of graft harvesting with RIA tube assembly mounted on RIA shaft and attached filter collecting the harvested bone graft.

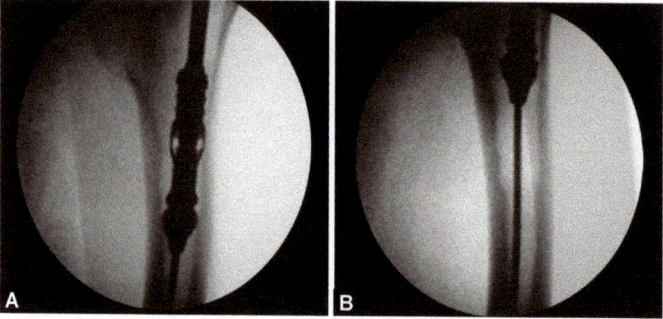

Fig. 14.13A and B: (A) Shows RIA reamer (13.5 mm) in process of reaming the medullary cavity (12 mm) with back and forth action; (B) Shows the reamed inside cortex depicting the enlarged width of medullary canal after reaming proximally.

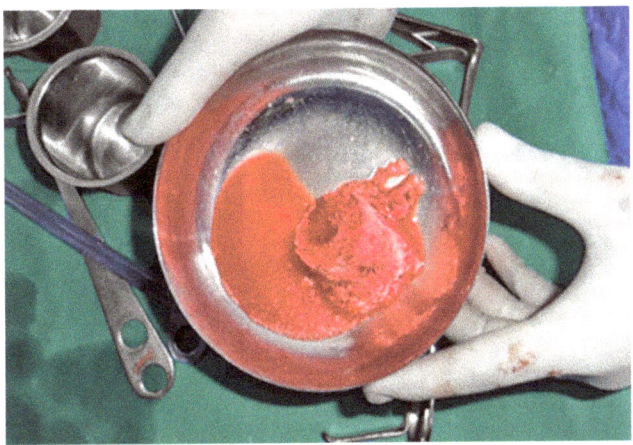

Fig. 14.14: Reamings collected in bowl.

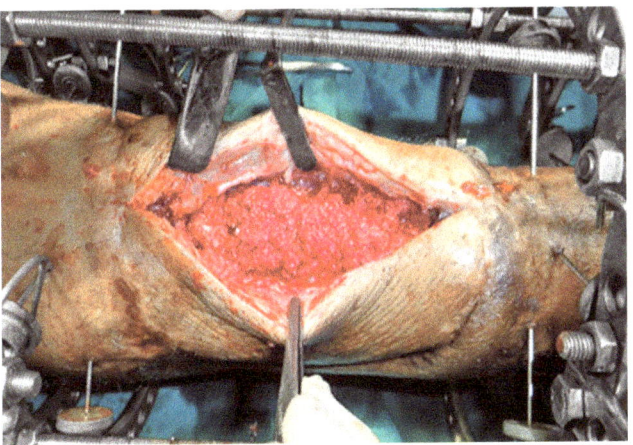

Fig. 14.15: Reamer/Irrigator/Aspirator device harvested graft filling 6 inch bone defect.

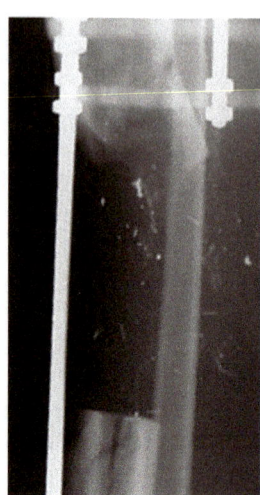

Fig. 14.16: Initial X-ray.

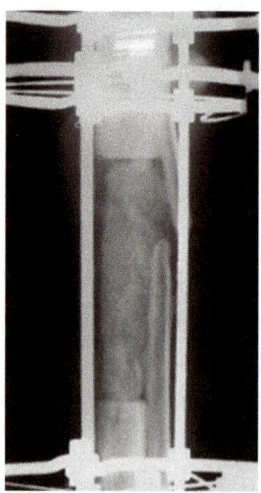

Fig. 14.17: X-ray after RIA grafting, immediate postoperative.

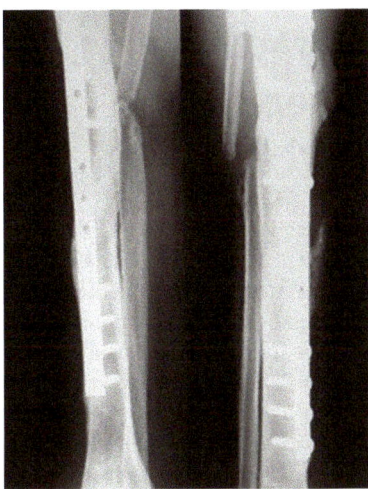

Fig. 14.18: Ilizarov frame removed and plate fixation done for further consolidation.

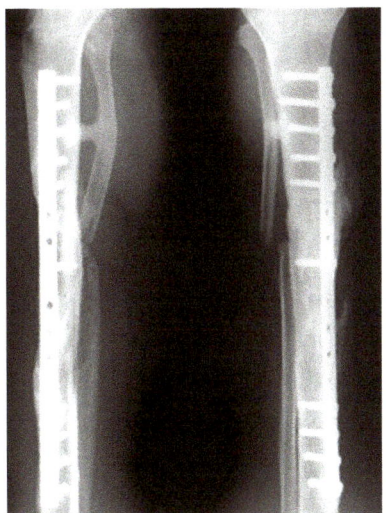

Fig. 14.19: Follow-up X-ray at 4 years shows complete consolidation.

J Nail Fixation for Surgical Neck Humerus Fractures in Elderly Osteoporotic Bones

Chapter 15

RM Chandak

Proximal humerus fracture (Fig. 15.1) typically occurs in elderly patients commonly associated with osteoporosis and is usually managed with open reduction and internal fixation, with locking plate technique with PHILOS plate. Despite the application of modern plate technology, complications remain common after fixation of proximal humeral fracture in elderly patients. Varus deformity, intra-articular hardware, screw loosening, avascular necrosis, and loss of head contour are often responsible for poor results in some patients. J nail fixation (Figs. 15.2 to 15.3) being closed method, providing 3 point fixation, avoids many of

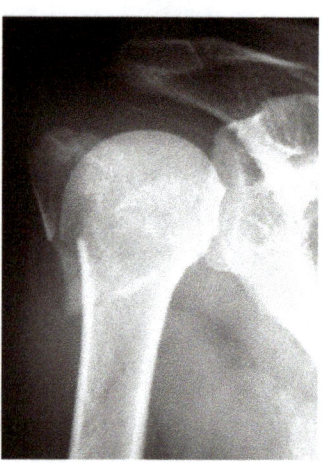

Fig. 15.1: Three part valgus impacted fracture.

Chapter 15: J Nail Fixation for Surgical Neck Humerus...

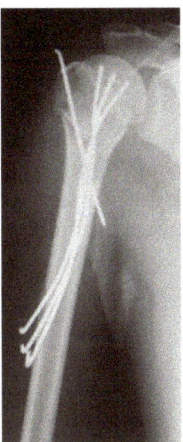

Fig. 15.2: Note the entry point from anteromedial surface of humerus in a case of varus displaced fracture pattern.

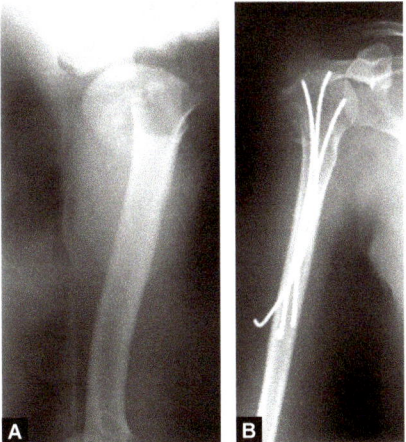

Figs. 15.3A and B: Construct for valgus impacted.

the complications associated with open PHILOS plate fixation and avoids surgical devascularization of fragments.

J nail fixation also has the advantage of being almost a closed method without the disadvantage of muscle transfixation. The procedure is simple and involves minimum invasion of soft tissue. Shoulder and elbow function is not impeded because the nails are inserted just below the distal part of the deltoid insertion. This surgical technique is described pictorially and with X-rays with figures from (Figs. 15.4 to 15.9).

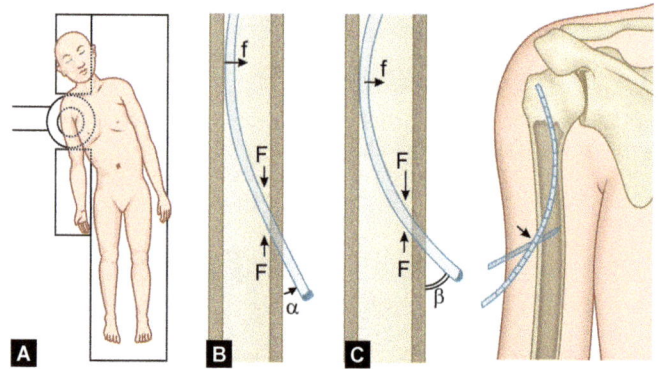

Figs. 15.4A to C: (A) Supine position on table, with Backlite extension board for obtaining AP and axial views; (B) Showing oblique J nail trajectory; (C) Shows multiple point fixation.

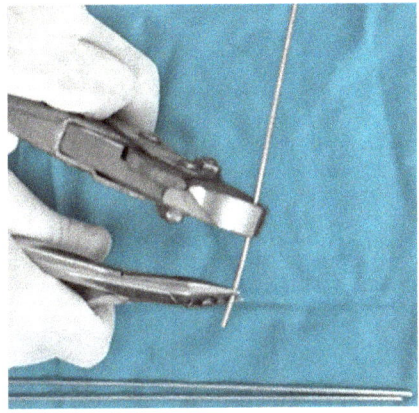

Fig. 15.5: J nail preparation on trolley.

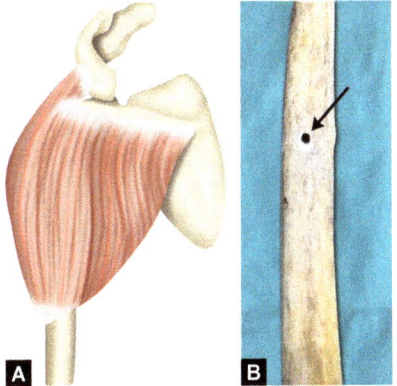

Figs. 15.6A and B: Entry point for J nail just below deltoid insertion, at mid arm level on anterolateral surface of humerus.

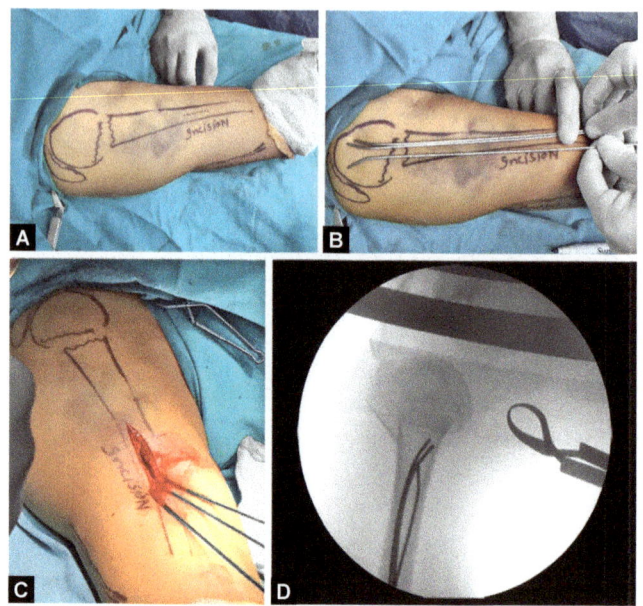

Figs. 15.7A to D: (A) Surface marking of fracture surgical neck humerus; (B) Anticipated trajectory mapping of J nail; (C) Shows incision and three J nails in three different entry holes; (D) Entry point with 2.5 mm K-wire and hammered up to fracture site as seen on C-arm image.

PLANNING J NAIL PLACEMENT

Oblique entry point drilled with 2.5 mm K-wire.

For Entry Point

- Midshaft 3 cm incisions.
- Drilling as parallel to humerus as possible (self-loading—collet function drill), try to negotiate into the medullary cavity.

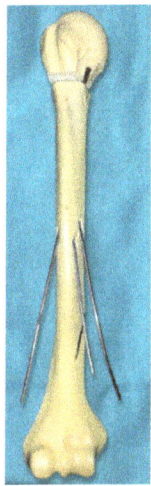

Fig. 15.8: Note the oblique entry point.

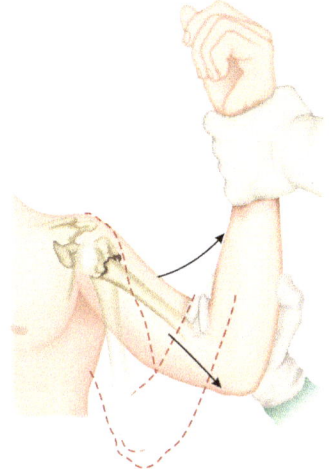

Fig. 15.9: Shaft pulled out; abduction, external rotation and traction.

Reduction Maneuver

In varus displaced fractures pins are to be inserted on either side of anterior border.

Advantages (Figs. 15.10 to 15.14)

- Faster and good healing.
- No varus.
- Good construct.
- Enhanced relative stability.
- Good callus formation.

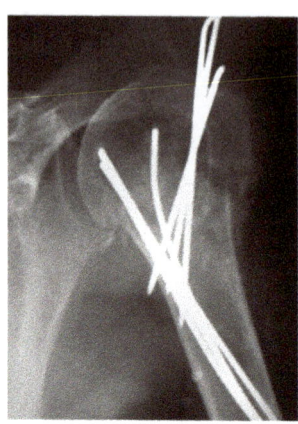

Fig. 15.10: Shows good callus as early as 6 weeks.

CASE I

Preoperative

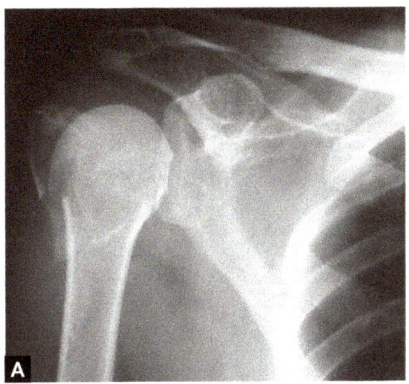

Postoperative

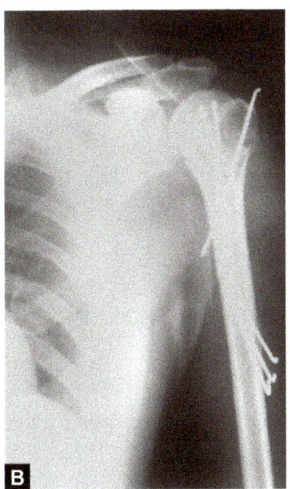

Figs. 15.11A and B: (A) Valgus impacted three part fracture; (B) Note good healing; Look at greater trochanter (GT) in position.

CASE II

Preoperative

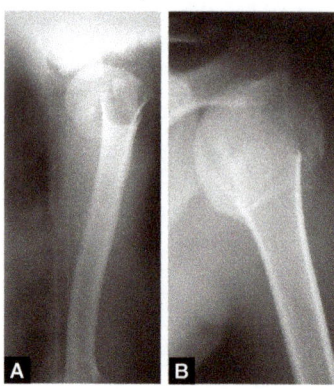

Postoperative

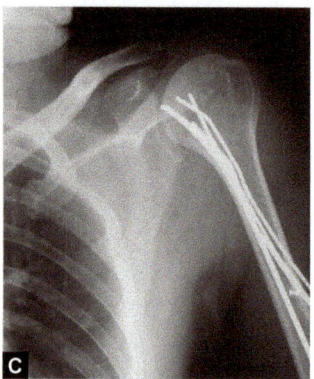

Figs. 15.12A to C: (A and B) Varus displaced fracture; (C) J nail in position.

CASE III

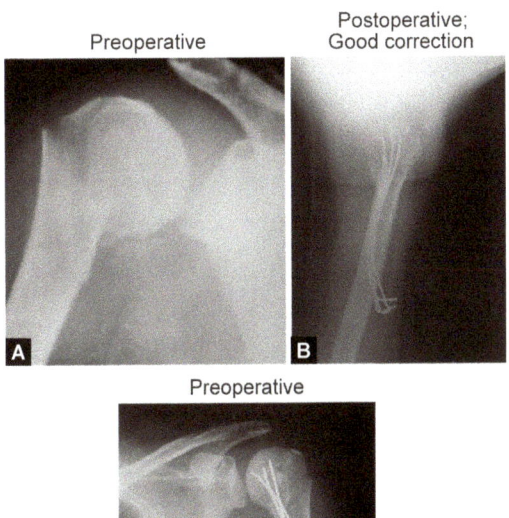

Figs. 15.13A to C: (A) Note varus displaced fracture pattern; (B and C) Postoperative image showing good reduction achieved.

Nota Bene

Benefits of arching J nail technique (multiple point fixation) rather than a straight K-wire:
- Avoids unsafe zone for drilling.
- Maintains reduction.
- Maintains head shaft angle.
- Does not easily back out.
- It is biological.

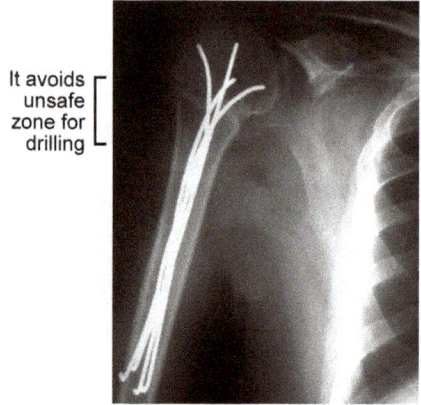

Fig. 15.14: Avoids varus, note good fanning.

# Screw Intramedullary Nail in Adult Forearm Fractures: New Concept

Chapter 16

Wasudeo Gadegone

INTRODUCTION

The restoration of radial bow, reconstruction of the radioulnar joints, and early commencement of movements are vital to gain excellent forearm function which can be accomplished by closed locked intramedullary nail but procedure is technically demanding. The screw intramedullary device which anchors to the metaphyseal bone by the wide screw head at the end of the nail and the distal beveled end of the nail aids in fracture reduction and helps in engaging in the subchondral area of the bone which has given consistently good to excellent results.

THE DESIGN OF THE SCREW INTRAMEDULLARY NAIL

The screw intramedullary nail (Titanium or steel) is a smooth circular implant and is available in diameters of 2 mm, 2.5 mm, and 3 mm with beveled tip. A threaded head, blended with the nail, is positioned at the end of nail held in place by circular running notch located on the end of nail shaft. This design allows the self-cutting thread to be advanced and screwed in with a screwdriver. The nail is sufficiently elastic to bend as it traverses the canal from the point of insertion and resilient enough to spring back in the curvature when finally seated (Fig. 16.1).

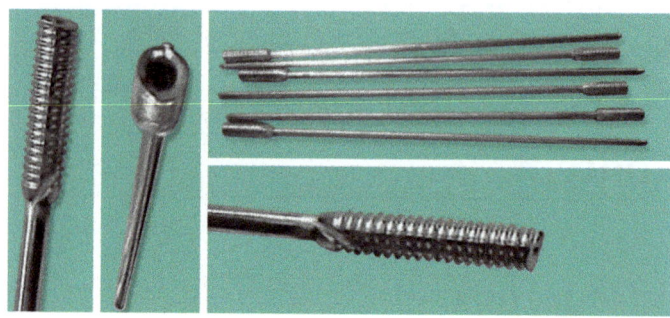

Fig. 16.1: Screw IM clavicle nails of various sizes with close up view of the head portion of the nail.

SURGICAL TECHNIQUE

Preoperative Preparation

X-ray of affected forearm is taken in anteroposterior (AP) and lateral view to evaluate the fracture displacement, assessment of the medullary canal diameter, and to select the length of the nail.

Position of the Patient and Reduction of Fracture

Under brachial block, patient is placed on the side of fracture table with elbow post for counter traction to freely visualize the bone under C-arm.

On fracture table with elbow post for counter traction and manual traction by assistant holding the hand of the patient or applying a forearm distractor by manipulation, the fracture is reduced by closed method (Figs. 16.2A and B).

In difficulty of closed reduction, fragments are manipulated by percutaneous K-wire. The reduction is checked under C-arm.

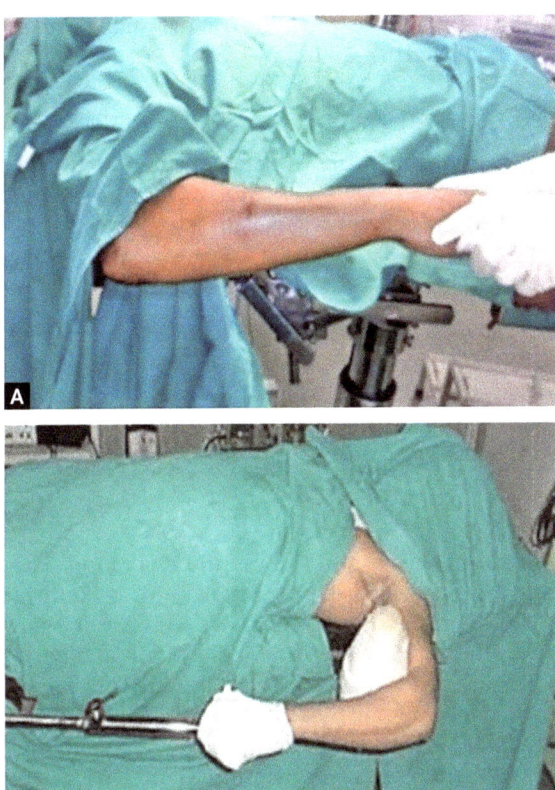

Figs. 16.2A and B: (A) Manual traction; (B) Traction with forearm distractor.

Which Bone First to Nail

Usually one bone reduction is achieved by manipulation. Nailing is first done of reduced bone as this might help in restoring length and alignment of the forearm. We prefer to address antegrade nailing of the ulna fracture first due to its subcutaneous position. After that, reduction of the second bone is attempted. We nailed the ulna antegrade first, providing a more stable forearm for retrograde nailing of the radius.

Entry Point

The ulna is approached from the radial side of the olecranon tip or tip of the olecranon and the radius is entered preferably through the styloid process or radial to Lister's tubercle.

Reaming of the Canal

The ulnar canal proximal to fracture is gradually reamed starting with 2.5 mm reamer to maximum possible size. Reaming of the canal distal to the fracture site is attempted by reducing the fracture. Reaming of the radius canal is done in cases of very narrow canal up to isthmus.

Ulna Nailing (Figs. 16.3A to F)

Small incision is given at the tip of the olecranon. The hole is created with the help of straight awl and is confirmed in C-arm. Reaming is done. A 2.5 mm or 3 mm elastic screw nail is introduced through the tip of the olecranon and negotiated across the fracture and lastly screwing is done with screwdriver till it reaches subchondral bone. If there is difficulty in reduction or loss of reduction while passing nail, K-wire manipulation of fracture fragments is done to help negotiation of nail through fracture site.

Radius Nailing (Figs. 16.4A to D)

In the radius fracture, bowing of the radius can be achieved by proper contouring of the nail. This is to maintain the normal rotation of radius on the ulna. The radius is entered preferably through the styloid process. A small incision is given over the ulnar side of the radial styloid process. Curved awl is passed first perpendicular to bone and then directed toward the radius canal. Entry of awl is confirmed in C-arm. Entry portal is enlarged

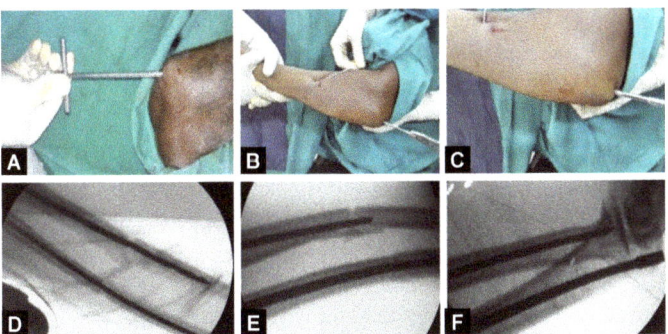

Figs. 16.3A to F: Ulna nailing procedure. (A) Entry point; (B) K-wire to hold the reduction; (C) Reaming of canal; (D to F) Reaming and introduction of nail.

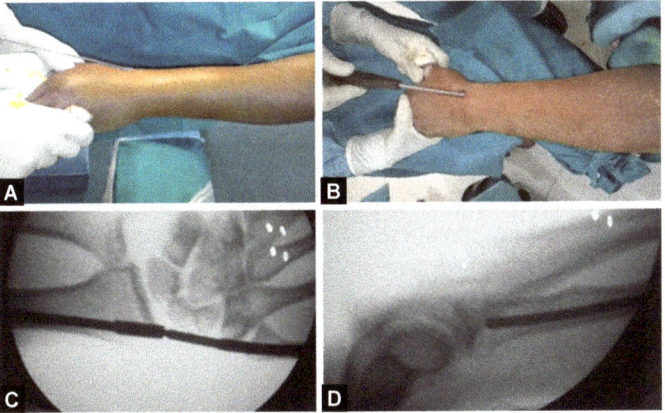

Figs. 16.4A to D: Radius nailing procedure. (A) Reduction; (B) Entry point; (C and D) Introduction of nail.

gradually up to 4 mm to accept a larger diameter base of the nail. Up to 3-mm diameter nails need only general prebending as they are flexible enough to conform to the bows. A 2.5 mm or 3 mm prebent elastic screw intramedullary nail is then introduced through the window of the radius and negotiated till it reaches the subchondral bone of radial head crossing the fracture. The stability is assessed while the nail is *in situ* and checked under the C-arm.

When to do Open Reduction?

If closed reduction is not possible, mini open reduction can be done to reduce the fracture and negotiate the nail and when bone grafting is needed. It is very important that the screw end is buried into the metaphyseal region as the bone imparts stability and which shall prevent nail migration and irritation of the overlying structures.

When to do Stack Nailing?

If the construct is unstable, and translation at fracture site after first nail then we advocate stacking the fracture site with an additional nail through the radius or ulna by creating a nail entry point adjacent to the previously passed nail. Due to stacking of nails, the construct fills in the medullary cavity and provides excellent rotational stability and this also eliminates need for a cast or brace. The flexible nature of the nails allows for restoration of the radial bow and interosseous space this was evident in the following images (Figs. 16.5A to C) (Figs. 16.6A to D).

Rehabilitation

An above-elbow cast is given for a period of 6 weeks. Active finger movements are started immediately after the operation. The cast is removed after 4 to 6 weeks depending on the stability of construct and the radiographs are obtained. Physiotherapy for elbow and wrist is initiated. When fracture union (defined as radiographic union with no pain or motion with manual stressing of the fracture) is evident, return to full activities (including sports) at 3 months.

Screw elastic intramedullary nail is an implant with a short learning curve. It effectively controls both rotatory forces and the

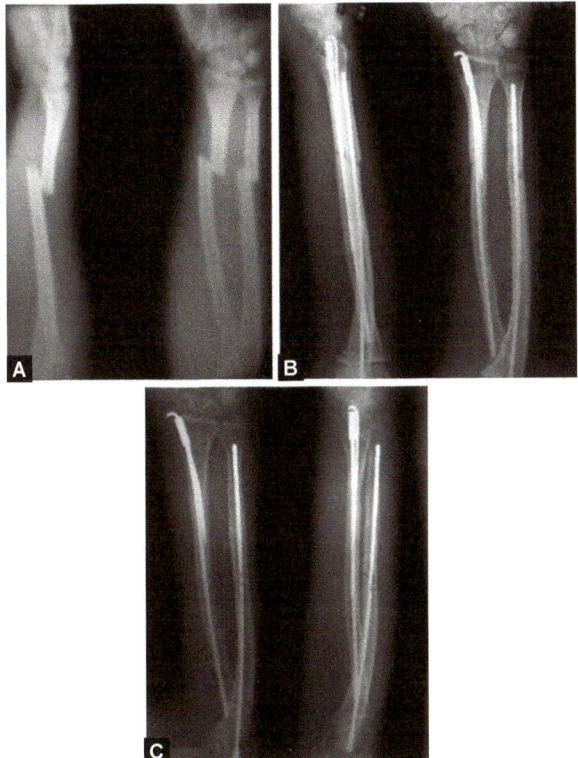

Figs. 16.5A to C: (A) Anteroposterior and lateral radiographs of both bone forearm with wrist in a; (B) Postoperative radiographs after nailing, which required a stacked additional nail; (C) Union of fracture. Stacked nailing and restoration of radial bow.

migration of the nail instrumentation. This implant addresses the biological concept of the fracture healing.

PITFALLS AND PEARLS

- *Which bone to fix first?*: The bone that is reduced easily by closed manipulation, if not radius is first.

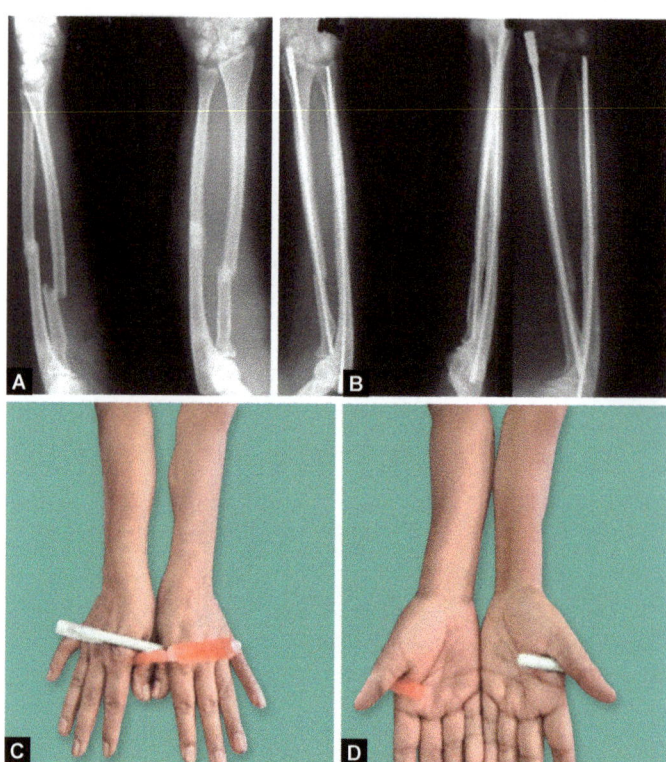

Figs. 16.6A to D: (A) Anteroposterior and lateral radiographs of both bone forearm with wrist; (B) Postoperative radiographs after nailing; (C) Union of fracture; (D) Clinical photograph. Close intramedullary nailing with good union and full function.

- *When to do mini open reduction?*: After 2–3 attempts at reduction with the help of reduction tools like K-wire; if not successful, limited open reduction should be tried.
- *In disparity of canal diameter*: The second nail should be passed by the side of first nail till it stacks in diaphysis.

- *Injury to superficial radial nerve*: It should be avoided at the time of entry point incision for radius by locating the surface anatomy.
- Before you close the wound, distraction and malrotation must be checked.
- A 2–3 mm end of nail should be outside the bone for easy removal.
- Fracture distraction and iatrogenic comminution can be prevented by preoperative canal assessment and insertion of proper size nail.
- Holding a good fracture reduction during the reaming of the intramedullary canal and insertion of nail, prebending of nail before inserting helps restore and maintain the anatomy to an acceptable limit of 10° in any plane.

SUGGESTED READING

1. Gadegone W, Salphale YS, Lokhande V. Screw elastic intramedullary nail for the management of adult forearm fractures. Indian J Orthop. 2012;46(1):65-70.
2. Gadegone WM, Salphale Y, Magarkar D. Percutaneous osteosynthesis of Galeazzi fracture-dislocation. Indian J Orthop. 2010;44(4):448-52.
3. Sage FP, Smith H. Medullary fixation of forearm fractures. J Bone Joint Surg Am. 1959;39:91-8.
4. Street DM. Intramedullary forearm nailing. Clin Orthop Relat Res. 1986;212:219-30.
5. Visna P, Beitl E, Pilný J, et al. Interlocking nailing of forearm fractures. Acta Chir Belg. 2008;108(3):333-8.

Chapter 17

Humerus Nailing in Lateral Position

Wasudeo Gadegone

INTRODUCTION

With advent of good designs of nails, straight and angled in the arena of treatment for fractures from surgical neck of humerus to approximately 5 cm above the olecranon fossa, nailing is gaining popularity in recent literature. Beach chair is the preferred position by many, but there is always difficulty in distal locking by free hand technique due to rounded smooth anatomy of anterior distal humerus and fear of neurovascular complications in both anteroposterior (AP) and lateromedial locking.

The aim of this chapter is to demonstrate the utility of lateral position in ease of nailing all types of humerus fractures. The technique and illustrations below describe the positioning of patient, image intensifier, and free hand posteroanterior distal locking.

OPERATIVE TECHNIQUE

Patient Positioning

Patient is placed on radiolucent orthopedic table in contralateral to lateral decubitus position with 10–15° posterior sag of ipsilateral shoulder. Patient's body is secured with well-padded side supports over the sacrum and pubis, soft cushioning at all bony prominences, and appropriate head-neck elevation for adequate airway access (Fig. 17.1).

Positioning of the patient, surgeon, assistant, image intensifier, and the anesthetist with his machine at a predefined place is the key in execution of the surgery. The surgeon stands

Chapter 17: Humerus Nailing in Lateral Position

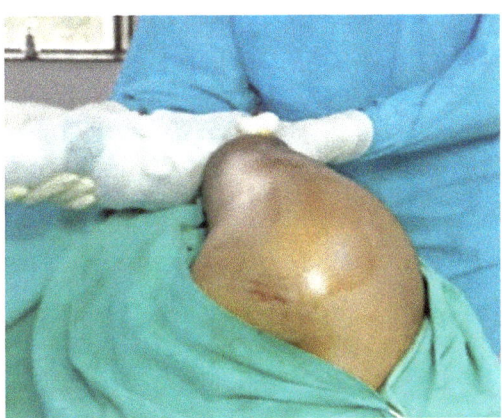

Fig. 17.1: Lateral position of patient.

at the head end of the patient's shoulder and assistant stands opposite to the surgeon at posterior aspect of the patient holding the arm at forearm and elbow. The assistant has a pivotal role in achieving and maintaining reduction with traction and manipulation of the arm with viewing images in all planes during the procedure. Image intensifier is placed in transverse plane giving unobstructed anteroposterior view from shoulder to elbow at all times. Viewing in different planes is usually achieved by rotating the image intensifier or changing of position of shoulder arm and elbow rotation (Figs. 17.2A to F).

Reduction of Fracture and Entry Point

Patient is placed in the lateral position. A small 2 cm skin incision from the anterolateral edge of the acromion is given and subcutaneous tissue sharply incised. Deltoid muscle is split along the raphe followed by incising and/or partially resecting the subdeltoid bursa. The supraspinatus tendon is incised in line with its fibers with a pointed scalpel blade.

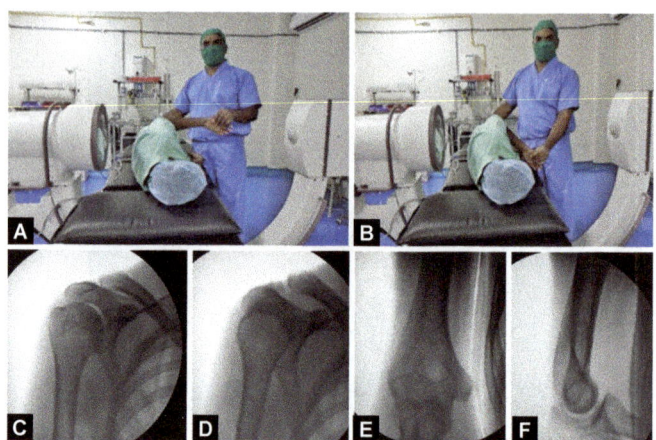

Figs. 17.2A to F: C-arm position and images of proximal and distal humerus reduction of fracture. (A) Lateral position; (B) Position of assistant; (C and D) C-arm Images of shoulder; (E and F) C-arm images of elbow.

Fracture is reduced by using traction, varus/valgus, and rotational force applied manually. Entry point is located at the lateral edge of articular surface in AP plane and at center of humeral head in lateral plane with a 3-mm Steinmann pin and confirmed under C-arm image.

The entry point is enlarged with bone awl and a 2.5 mm guidewire is passed through the correct entry point and guidewire is passed across the fracture site.

Reaming of the Canal

Reaming of the canal is carried out sequentially through the fracture site into the distal medullary canal up to 1 cm proximal to olecranon fossa (Figs. 17.3A to D).

Insertion of Nail

The appropriate size and length of the humerus nail is inserted with slightly rotating movements down to the fracture line. The

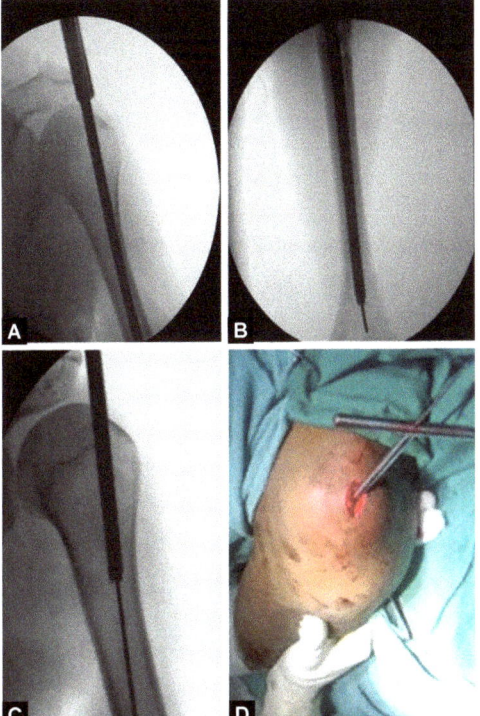

Figs. 17.3A to D: Reaming. Sequential reaming over the guidewire.

fracture site firmly held by the assist to avoid movements at the fracture site which helps in the prevention of injury to the radial nerve. The nail is passed across the fracture site and final seating of the nail is done in distal metaphysis with gentle blows after accurate control of rotation.

Proximal Locking

Proximal locking is done with help of jig. Number of locking screws and their position depends on the fracture configuration

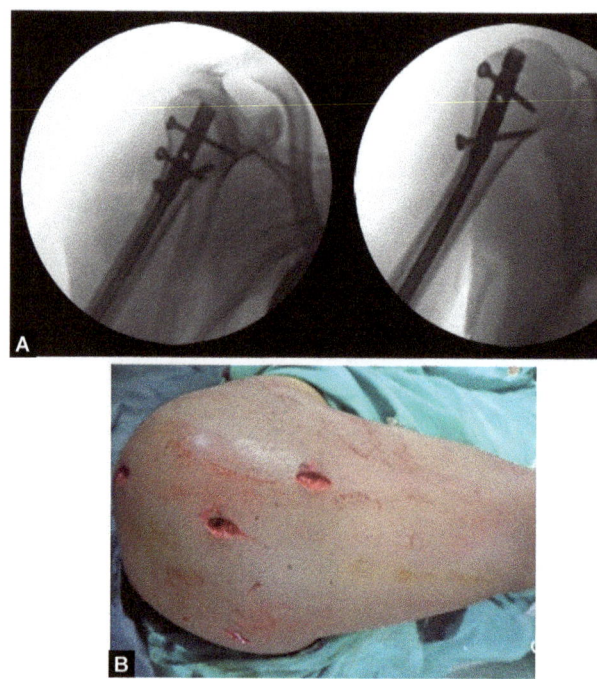

Figs. 17.4A and B: Proximal locking.

and location. At least two proximal bolts are considered sufficient for shaft fractures and multiple angled locking with maximum bolts is required for proximal and metaphyseal fracture. If gapping is evident at fracture site, elbow is stroked gently to achieve compression or first distal locking and extraction blows shall achieve compression at fracture site. Check the nail is subarticular and then do proximal locking (Figs. 17.4A and B).

Distal Locking

During free hand distal locking, the patient's arm rests on his or her body and the forearm is rested on the anterior pelvic

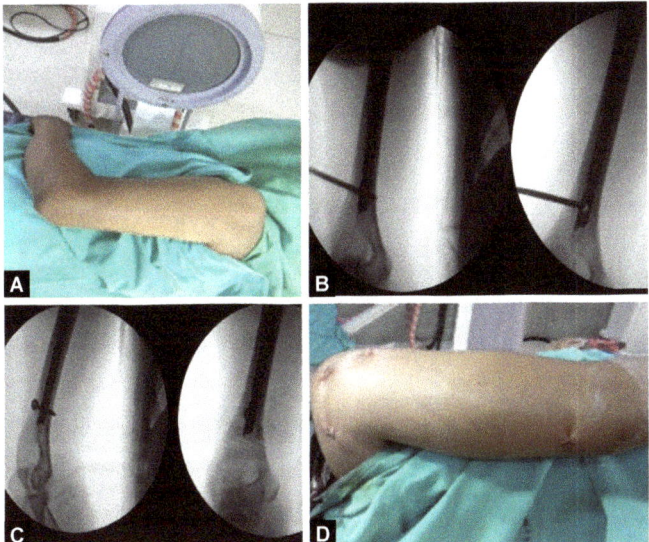

Figs. 17.5A to D: Distal locking in lateral position.

support on sterile padding. By changing the amount of padding, arm rotation can be adjusted to give a perfect view of the distal locking hole. Once distal interlock holes appear as perfect circles in AP view, a small stab incision is taken on posterior part of the lower arm. The hole is located with a 3 mm K-wire and posterior cortex is perforated. The K-wire is replaced by 3.5 mm drill bit and further cortex is drilled and locking is done with 3.9 mm appropriate length screw. Posterior surface of humerus is flat with less musculature, hence positioning of drill and locking is easy. Implant position, fracture reduction is checked in both planes and the zig removed (Figs. 17.5A to D).

Wounds are copiously irrigated and closed in layers. Postoterative images are taken to check the reduction, placement of nail and screws (Figs. 17.6A and B).

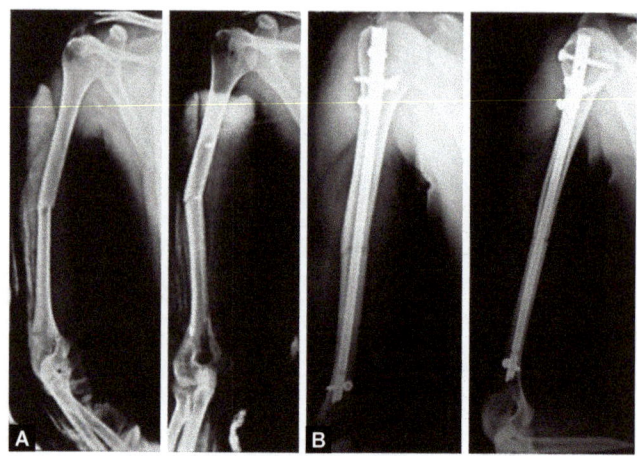

Figs. 17.6A and B: Diaphyseal fracture humerus. (A) Preoperative X-ray and (B) Postoperative X-ray.

Rehabilitation

Immediate postoperative arm is placed in a sling pouch. Patients are encouraged to start finger, wrist, and elbow movements once the anesthesia weans off. Gentle pendulum exercises, shoulder shrugs, and static exercises are begun once pain free.

The humeral fracture fixation with locked intramedullary nailing in lateral position offers an appealing solution.

ADVANTAGES OF LATERAL POSITION

The humerus nailing is advantageous in lateral position as:
- Entry point location is easy extending the shoulder without changing the position of C-arm.
- Unobstructed views from shoulder to elbow are possible without repeated change in positioning of image intensifier.
- Manipulation of the fracture and the limb is possible with ease.

- Posteroanterior distal locking proves to be the biggest advantage of this position as found by easier hole location, no slippage on flat posterior surface, and no risk of neurovascular damage.

PEARLS AND PITFALLS

- Entry point depends on the design of nail.
- Incision through the supraspinatus in line with its fibers.
- Before proximal or distal locking care must be taken for exact placement of tip of the subarticular nail.
- No distraction at the fracture site.
- Patient may experience tingling and numbness in a lower down contralateral limb.
- True lateral picture is not possible in this position.
- Firm support at the fracture site while reduction and reaming to avoid injury to radial nerve.
- Early mobilization of shoulder to avoid adhesions and stiffness.

SUGGESTED READING

1. Blyth MJ, Macleod CM, Asante DK, et al. Iatrogenic nerve injury with the Russell–Taylor humeral nail. Injury. 2003;34(3):227-8.
2. Gadegone WM, Salphale YS. Antegrade rush nailing for fractures of humeral shaft: an analysis of 200 cases with an average follow-up of 1 year. Eur J Orthop Surg & Traumatol. 2008;18(2):93-9.
3. Garnavos C. Diaphyseal humeral fractures and intramedullary nailing: Can we improve outcomes? Indian J Orthop. 2011;45(3):208-15.
4. Noger M, Berli MC, Fasel JH, et al. The risk of injury to neurovascular structures from distal locking screws of the Unreamed Humeral Nail (UHN): a cadaveric study. Injury. 2007;38(8):954-7.

Chapter 18

Screw Intramedullary Fixation of Displaced Clavicle Fractures

Wasudeo Gadegone

INTRODUCTION

Surgical stabilization may be indicated in cases with completely displaced fractures (gap of >20 mm), potential skin perforation, shortening of clavicle by more than 20 mm, neurovascular injury, and floating shoulder injury. Intramedullary (IM) nailing has been successfully used by few authors but has complications like nail migration and nonunion.

This chapter describes the technique of using the screw intramedullary nail for displaced clavicle fracture. The screw nail, which anchors to the metaphyseal bone by the wide screw head at the end of the nail, results into a stable construct which prevents migration of nail and produces consistently good to excellent results.

IMPLANT DESIGN

Screw elastic intramedullary nail is made of titanium or steel and is available in diameters of 2 mm, 2.5 mm, and 3 mm. The nails are 5–6 cm in length, with screw portion of 10 mm length and 4.5 mm in diameter. The screw head is of 3.5 mm size where the appropriate screwdriver fits. The nail is made of either steel or titanium and is sufficiently elastic to bend as it traversed the canal from the point of insertion and resilient enough to spring back in the curvature when finally seated. However it is still rigid enough to withstand the torsional, rotational, and angulatory forces. Nail has a beveled tip at one end and a threaded head positioned at the other. This design allows the self-cutting thread to be advanced and screwed in with a 3.5 mm screwdriver (Fig. 18.1).

The distal beveled end of the nail aids in fracture reduction and helps in engaging in the flat area of the bone, thereby imparting stability. A special type of nail holding instrument or chuck is mandatory to firmly hold the screw nail.

STEP-BY-STEP DESCRIPTION OF SURGICAL TECHNIQUE

Preoperative Planning

X-ray of affected clavicle is taken in anteroposterior, caudal, and cranial view to evaluate the fracture displacement, assessment of the medullary canal diameter, and length of the nail (Fig. 18.2).

Position of the Patient

Operative procedure is carried out under interscalene block or general anesthesia. Affected shoulder is elevated by a bolster so that clavicle becomes more prominent. This position also helps to restore length and increase exposure of the clavicle. The procedure is performed under fluoroscopic guidance.

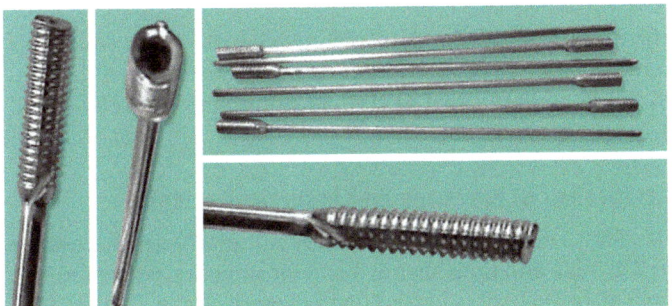

Fig. 18.1: Screw clavicle nails of various sizes with close up view of the head portion of the nail.

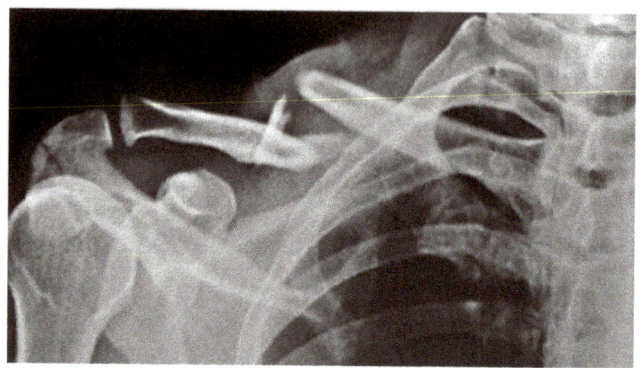

Fig. 18.2: Displaced clavicle fracture.

Surgical Approach

A 1-cm skin incision is made over medial end of clavicle just lateral to sternoclavicular joint. The insertion point is made approximately 1 cm lateral to the sternoclavicular joint. A hole is created in the anterior cortex with a straight pointed awl and the entry portal is then enlarged with a curved awl directing toward axis of the medullary cavity.

Reaming of the Canal

The reaming of canal is done with sequential reamer and then a screw elastic nail of appropriate diameter and length is inserted in the medullary canal of clavicle with a universal chuck and T-handle or screw inserter.

Reduction of Fracture and Insertion of Nail

Usually 2.5 mm screw intramedullary nail attached to the inserter or T-handle and tip is slightly bend for smooth passage through the canal. The nail is passed first perpendicular with oscillating movements; the nail is advanced until it reaches the fracture site. With the help of percutaneously placed towel clips, fracture

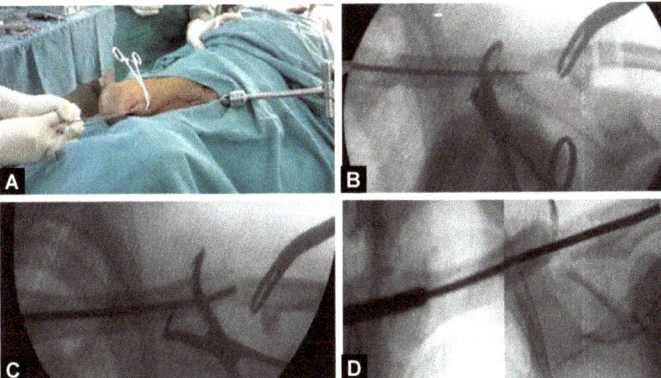

Figs. 18.3A to D: (A) Negotiation of nail; (B) Reduction; (C) Negotiation of nail through fracture; (D) Final placement.

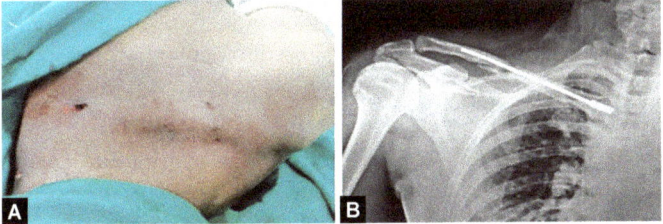

Figs. 18.4A and B: (A) Mostly closed surgery; (B) Final sitting of screw in metaphysis.

fragments are approximated by lifting and maneuvering under C-arm (Figs. 18.3A to D).

The reduction is checked in image-intensifier and then the nail is advanced through the fracture site till it reaches distal end of clavicle. Generally nail can be negotiated 1 cm short of acromioclavicular joint (Figs. 18.4A and B).

If Closed Reduction Fails

If closed reduction is unsuccessful, an additional skin incision is made at fracture site for open reduction of the fragments.

Although clavicle is S-shaped, tip of the nail is curved which helps the surgeon to pass the elastic nail into distal fragment. After adequate engagement of the distal fragment, the medial end of screw nail is screwed in the metaphyseal region of the medial end of clavicle and skin closed over it.

Rehabilitation

Postoperatively arm pouch sling is given for 3 weeks and gentle pendulum exercises of the shoulder are allowed as per pain tolerance immediately after surgery.

ADVANTAGES

The use of an intramedullary device carries advantages of a smaller incision, less soft tissue dissection, load sharing fixation with relative stability that encourages callus formation. It should also be noted that removal of nail as additional surgical procedure requires only small incision and short duration of hospital stay.

PITFALLS AND CHALLENGES

- Care should be taken while opening the medial cortex otherwise injury to the lungs and vessels may occur because of slipping of awl over the smooth anterior cortex.
- Too medial entry shall cause irritation and prominence at sternoclavicular joint.
- Screw should be buried inside the metaphysis leaving near about 3–4 mm out of bone for easy removal.
- In a comminuted fracture, both ends must be well secured in the bone otherwise axial compression may result into shortening of clavicle and prominence of the screw.
- Diameter less than 2 mm of the nail does not give support; hence in narrow canal, nailing should not be attempted.
- Failure of reduction after 2–3 attempts, it is better to do mini open reduction.
- Be careful while negotiating tip through fracture under C-arm to avoid injury to underneath neurovascular bundle.

SUGGESTED READING

1. Frigg A, Rillmann P, Perren T, et al. Intramedullary nailing of clavicular midshaft fractures with the titanium elastic nail: problems and complications. Am J Sports Med. 2009;37:352-9.
2. Gadegone WM, Lokhande V. Screw Intramedullary Elastic Nail Fixation in Midshaft Clavicle Fractures: A Clinical Outcome in 36 Patients. Indian J Orthop. 2018;52(3):322-7.
3. Hussain N, Sermer C, Prusick PJ, et al. Intramedullary nailing versus plate fixation for the treatment displaced midshaft clavicular fractures: a systematic review and meta-analysis. Sci Rep. 2016;6:34912.
4. Rehm K, Andermahr J, Jubel A. Intramedullary nailing of midclavicular fractures with an elastic titanium nail. Eur J Traum Emerg Surg. 2005;31:409-16.

Index

Page numbers followed by *f* refer to figure.

A

Acetabular tuberculosis 67
Acetabulum
    arthritic changes in 86*f*
    osteoarthritis of 86
    posterior column of 69*f*
Align fracture 98*f*
American Society for Bone and Mineral Research 9
Ankle
    exercises using shoe 2*f*
    fracture 168, 179*f*
    joint 180*f*
Antibiotic
    bone cement block 195*f*
    cement spacer 194*f*
    spacer flap 195*f*
Austin Moore
    prosthesis 86, 88
    removal 86
Auto cancellous graft 50*f*
Avascular necrosis 69, 126, 162, 162*f*, 202
    fibula intrafemoral 163*f*
    hips 79*f*
Avulsion 187*f*
    sprain, chronic 77

B

Big thick capsule 86
Bisphosphonate-induced fractures 9
Black metallic debris 84*f*
Blunt injury 6
Bone
    biopsies 11
    densitometry 124
    dissection around 38*f*
    formation 112*f*
    fragment, fixation of 134*f*
    graft 198*f*
        secondary 41
    ingrowth 90*f*
    large chunk of 133*f*
    morphogenetic protein 12
    nonunions, long 162
    removal of 89*f*
Bony
    erosion, nonspecific 82*f*
    in growth 89*f*, 99*f*
    projection, small 74*f*
Broken nail 96
    after removal 110*f*
    extractor reamer 101*f*
    removal 96
        instrument 102*f*, 109*f*
    with non-union 159*f*
Broken screw
    bone formation around periphery of 112*f*
    removal 102
Butterfly fragment 25*f*

C

Calcium 125*f*, 127
    supplements 80
Canal
    diameter, disparity of 220
    obliteration of 15*f*
    reaming of 216, 224, 232
Capsulectomy 87*f*, 92
Capsulotomy 87*f*, 92
Carbide tip drill 106*f*
C-arm 15*f*
    image 224
Cerebrospinal fluid
    diversion, proximal 8
    leak 8
Chaput fracture 170
Coccydynia 33
Coccyx
    angulation of 33*f*
    flexion of 35*f*
    fracture of 33*f*
    injury of 34*f*
    pain in 33
Collateral ligament
    anterior medial 189*f*
    sutured medial 187*f*
Comminuted fracture 41, 44*f*, 45*f*, 47
    nailed 48*f*
    shaft femur 49*f*
Comminuted intertrochanteric fracture 26*f*
Corticocancellous graft 28*f*
Cruciate ligament, anterior 139, 140*f*

D

Deltoid ligament 169, 170
Depo-Medrol injection 77
    local 78*f*
Diaphyseal fracture humerus 228*f*
Displaced clavicle fracture 232*f*
    screw intramedullary fixation of 230
Distal locking 226, 227*f*
Dural tension, abnormal 35*f*
Dynamic compression plate 146*f*
Dynamic condylar screw 107
Dynamic hip screw 120, 123*f*, 165*f*
    removal 93

E

Elbow
    dislocation of 183, 185*f*
    function 204
    primary stabilizer of 191
Enchondroma 69, 71*f*

F

Femoral head, enchondroma of 69
Femoral nailing
    proximal 107
    short proximal 107*f*
Femoral neck, synovial herniation pit of 62
Femur 136
    canal 112*f*
    fibrous dysplasia of proximal 164*f*
    fragment of 49*f*
    hook plate, proximal 31*f*
    neck 27*f*
    neck fracture 116, 120
        conservative treatment of 120
        undisplaced 116
    plate, long 142*f*
        distal 149*f*

Fibrous dysplasia 164*f*
Fibula 143
  being trimmed 137*f*
  compound fracture of 192*f*
  distally 165*f*
  graft 50*f*, 143*f*, 144*f*, 153*f*, 154*f*
    harvested 136*f*
    harvesting, half 138*f*
    inserted intramedullary 139*f*
  inside joint 167*f*
    after collapse 166*f*
Fibular displacement, lateral 169*f*
Figure of 8 cerclage wire 134*f*
Fixing posterior malleolus 179
Forearm
  distractor, traction with 215*f*
  fractures, adult 213
Fracture 116, 128, 224
  and entry point, reduction of 223
  compression of 181*f*
  deterioration of 118*f*
  displaced 123*f*
  distal 52*f*, 53*f*
    humerus reduction of 224*f*
    part of 15*f*
  distraction 221
  fibula 170
  fragments, K-wire manipulation of 216
  healed with full function 51*f*
  healing of 12*f*, 13*f*, 158*f*, 161*f*
  hip 117, 117*f*
  insufficiency 127*f*
  pathological 164*f*
  posterior 182*f*
    wall 17*f*
  reduction of 214, 232
  shaft femur 25*f*
  site, union at 148*f*
  surgical neck humerus 146*f*, 206*f*
  transcervical 120
  transverse 15*f*, 52*f*
  type of 182*f*
    distal 53*f*
  undisplaced 120*f*, 122*f*
  union of 114*f*, 220*f*
  valgus impacted 121, 202*f*
    three part 209*f*
  with implant failure 93*f*
Fragment, large avulsed 132*f*

G

Gait
  correction 4
  training 5*f*
Grafted after curettage 72*f*
Grafting 65*f*
  fracture healed 43*f*
Greater trochanter 209*f*
  region 67

H

Head contour, loss of 202
Head of femur, idiopathic osteoporosis of 126, 127
Head of radius
  irreparable fracture of 183, 185*f*
  isolated fracture of 183
Hematoma 6*f*
  after blunt injury 6*f*
  formation 6
Hemiarthroplasty 27*f*
Herniation pit 66*f*
Hip
  area, pain in 63*f*
  fracture 123

pain 67
   minimal 70*f*
   replacement surgery 119*f*
   unexplained, pain in 82
Hook plate 32*f*
   to fix greater trochanter 32*f*
Hooked guidewire 97*f*
Humerus 136
   anteromedial surface of 203*f*
   fracture 20*f*
      proximal 202
   locking plate, proximal 30*f*
   philos plate, proximal 30*f*
   plate 95
      removal 95

I

Iatrogenic comminution 221
Idiopathic osteoporosis, changes of 80*f*
Iliac spine, anterior-inferior 77, 77*f*
Implant
   design 230
   infected 146*f*
   removal 86
Incision, posterior midline 133*f*
Infection 82
Inguinal area, pain in 73
Interfragmentary screw 23*f*, 25*f*
Interlock nailing 13*f*, 22*f*, 23*f*, 25*f*, 49*f*
Interosseous ligament 169, 170
Intra-articular hardware 202
Intramedullary fibula 136, 143*f*, 146*f*, 147*f*, 152*f*, 155*f*, 162*f*
   graft 136, 142*f*, 160*f*
      and plating 141*f*
   treated with 149*f*
   with plate 143*f*, 155*f*

Intramedullary nail 230
   treated with 141*f*
Intraoperative test 188*f*
Ipsilateral neck femur fracture 49*f*

J

J nail 210*f*
   anticipated trajectory mapping of 206*f*
   entry point for 205*f*
   fixation 202, 204
   placement, planning 206
   preparation on trolley 205*f*
Joint, displaced 175*f*

K

K nail 114, 115
   femur gauge 140*f*
   removal of embedded 114
Knee chest position 36*f*
K-wire 171, 190, 227
   to hold reduction 217*f*

L

Left hip, pain in 116, 117
Leg
   raising test, straight 58
   standing
      on affected 4*f*
      on normal 4*f*
Ligamentous components 169*f*
Ligaments
   heal properly 173*f*
   stitching 170*f*
Limp 73
Lister's tubercle 216
Locking nail with massive graft 145*f*
Locking plate 146*f*
   nice 145*f*

Loose coccyx piece, before surgery 39*f*
Loose prosthesis 87*f*

M

Malleolus fracture
  anterior posterior fixation of posterior 181*f*
  distal transverse medial 52
  medial 55*f*
  posterior 170, 179-81
Malunited ankle 55
Mantoux test 59
  negative 60*f*
Manual traction 215*f*
Massive cancellous bone graft 147*f*, 149*f*
Massive disk prolapse 58*f*, 59*f*
Massive grafting 145*f*
Measure fibula 140*f*
Medial cancellous graft 146*f*
  and plate 160*f*
Medial collateral ligament 183, 184, 187*f*
  sutured 189*f*
Medial fracture 182*f*
Medial ligament 170
Medial malleolus 52, 170
Medullary canal
  opening of blocked 16*f*
  stuffing thick nail 41
Medullary cavity, open up 138*f*
Mercedes-Benz sign 177*f*
Metaphyseal region 28*f*
Meticulous debridement 193*f*
Muscles, medial group of 187*f*

N

Nail 44
  broken
    part of 85*f*
    square 84*f*
  bypassing 22*f*
  distal end of 115*f*
  empty distal locking bolts of 99*f*
  extract broken 99*f*
  good designs of 222
  head portion of 214*f*, 231*f*
  in distraction 46*f*
  in long oblique fracture 25*f*
  insertion of 224, 232
  maintaining length 42*f*
  negotiation of 233*f*
  proximal part of 108*f*
Nailing
  length, closed 41*f*
  postoperative radiographs after 220*f*
Neck
  guidewire insertion in 17*f*
  screw removal 93
Nonunion 149*f*
  C-arm images of 143*f*
  distal femur 30*f*
  expected 160*f*
  femur 142*f*
  fracture humerus treated 141*f*
  intertrochanteric fracture 26, 31*f*
  of long bones
    management of 136
    treatment of 136
  site 139*f*
  with nail inside 141*f*

O

Olecranon
  post avulsion 129*f*
  tip of 128*f*, 132*f*
Osteoarthritis 86
Osteoporotic bones 202
Osteotomized neck 28*f*

P

Pain 73
Persistent sternoclavicular swelling 60*f*
Philos plate 147*f*
Plate 44
    bent over spoilt screw 105*f*
    broken 151*f*
    removal of 95
    with intramedullary fibula healed 141*f*
Post-pregnancy pain 79, 79*f*
Prolapsed intervertebral disc 58
Prosthesis, augment metaphyseal area of 28*f*
Pseudocapsule 86
Pseudo-joint, movements at 37*f*

R

Radial bow, restoration of 213
Radial nerve, superficial 221
Radioulnar joints, reconstruction of 213
Radius fracture 216
Radius nailing 216
    procedure 217*f*
Reamer/irrigator/aspirator system 192
Reaming medullary cavity 198*f*
Rectum 39*f*
Rectus femoris tendon 77, 77*f*
Right hip, pain in 82
Road traffic accident 192*f*

S

Sciatica 58*f*
Screw elastic intramedullary nail 230
Screw intramedullary nail 213
    design of 213
Screw loosening 202
Screw removal instruments, special 106*f*
Second surgery 159*f*
Segmental fracture
    humerus 141*f*
    tibia 24*f*
Sequestrectomy infection control 148*f*
Seroma
    cavity, suction drainage of 7*f*
    collection 6
Short wrist splint 1*f*
Shoulder
    exercises 3*f*
    function 204
    mobilizing exercises 3
Small incision 216
Smith-Peterson approach anterior incision 64*f*
Soft tissue 6
Square nail in situ 84*f*
Steinmann pin 100, 100*f*
Sternoclavicular joint, benign inflammation of 60*f*
Sternoclavicular swelling 59, 61*f*
Stress fracture 124, 125*f*
Subtrochanteric femur fracture 111*f*
Subtrochanteric fracture 107
Supination-pronation exercise 1
Supracondylar femur fracture, fixing accidental 29*f*
Surgical neck humerus fractures 202
Surgical technique, step-by-step description of 231
Syndesmosis 176*f*
Syndesmotic injury 168
    concepts of 173
    fixations, standard practice of 171*f*

typical 168*f*
Syndesmotic joint 168, 170, 173*f*
   open 177*f*
Syndesmotic region, stability to 180*f*
Synovial membrane 62, 66*f*
Synovial pit 66*f*

T

Tibia 136
   compound fracture of 192*f*
   distal 55*f*
Tibiofibular ligament
   anterior 170
      inferior 169
   attaches, posterior-inferior 180*f*
   posterior 170
      inferior 169
Tightrope fixation 174*f*
Tillaux fracture 170
Total hip replacement 16, 163*f*, 164*f*, 167*f*
   set 97
      long cement extractor forceps of revision 97*f*
Traction 22
Trochanteric fixation
   nail system 104
   replacement 27
Trochanteric osteotomy 89*f*

U

Ulna
   fracture, tip of 128
   nailing 216
      procedure 217*f*
Ulnar canal proximal to fracture 216

V

Vacuum assisted closure 193*f*, 194*f*
Valgus 224
   fracture 120*f*
   impacted, construct for 203*f*
Vancomycin 194*f*
Varus deformity 202
Varus displaced fracture 210*f*, 211*f*
   pattern 203*f*
   pins 207
Vitamin
   D 80, 125*f*
   D_3 126, 127

W

Waddling gait 124

X

X-ray elbow 128*f*

EU GSPR Authorised Reprsentative
Logos Europe, 9 rue Nicolas Poussin
1700, La Rochelle, France
Phone: +33 (0) 6 67 93 73 78
E-mail: contact@logoseurope.eu

www.ingramcontent.com/pod-product-compliance
Ingram Content Group UK Ltd.
Pitfield, Milton Keynes, MK11 3LW, UK
UKHW021146270226
468476UK00001B/6